Introduction

The Mediterranean diet is one of the healthiest and easiest diets in the world. It's full of vegetables, fruits, whole grains, nuts, legumes, fish, meat and cheese.

What's a Mediterranean Diet?

The Mediterranean diet is not so much a diet itself as a way of eating that is rich in flavor and variety. It consists of grains, vegetables, fruits, beans, oils, nuts, wine, and small portions of unprocessed meats like beef, chicken, pork and fish. The Mediterranean diet is based on the cuisines of countries bordering the Mediterranean Sea - Italy, Spain, France, Greece, and the countries of the Middle East. The difference between a Mediterranean diet and a traditional American diet is that the Mediterranean diet has more fruits and vegetables, fewer processed foods, smaller portions, and more fish and olive oil.

The Mediterranean diet originated in the 1950s, when scientists began studying the eating habits of people in the Mediterranean regions. They found that a diet rich in fruits, vegetables, fish and olive oil is linked with a lower risk of heart disease compared to a western diet, which consists of more processed foods and meat. Studies also found that the Mediterranean diet can lower the risk of some forms of cancer and can help treat diabetes, obesity, and hypertension. However, it is important to keep in mind that not all Mediterranean diets are healthy. Some Mediterranean diets include a lot of processed foods and ingredients high in saturated fat, such as butter, lard and red meat. A healthy Mediterranean diet focuses on fresh produce, whole grains, beans, and fish.

Below is a chart that shows highly nutritious foods straight from the Mediterranean. This Mediterranean food chart is a good way to help you determine if you're eating a healthy Mediterranean diet. Eating plenty of these nutritious foods is essential to good health, so you should make them a staple of your diet.

Vegetables and Fruits
✓   Olive oil. Eat it on bread and vegetables. Drizzle it on your pasta, rice or potatoes.
✓   Canned tomatoes. Boil, puree or grill in them.
✓   Artichokes. Grill them with olive oil and sea salt.
✓   Brussels sprouts. Puree, sauté or toss them with olive oil, garlic, and lemon juice.
✓   Tomatoes. Puree them or chop them up and use them as a topping on stuff like cheese and rice.
✓   Shrimp. Add them to pesto pasta or stir-fry.
✓   Lamb chops. Add capers and fresh mint to them and grill them.
✓   Feta cheese. Same as the lamb chops.
✓   Tuna. If it's canned, don't buy it.

Nuts and Legumes
✓   Chia seeds. Sprinkle them on just about anything.
✓   Chickpeas. Add to creme soups, salads, and sauces.
✓   Nuts. Nuts are high in fat, but they also contain many vitamins and minerals.
✓   Tahini. Packs a lot of protein for how small it is. Use it in salad dressings and sauces.

Grains and Beans
✓   Chickpeas.
✓   Lentils.
✓   Black beans.
✓   Garbanzo beans.
✓   Wheat berries.
✓   Bulgur.
✓   Brown rice.
✓   Quinoa.
✓   Farro.

Eggs and Dairy
✓   White beans.
✓   Whole-fat dairy.
✓   Oils.

Sauces, Dressings, and Condiments

✓   Caper sauce.
✓   Dill sauce.
✓   Lemon juice.
✓   Red wine vinegar.
✓   Extra-virgin olive oil.
✓   Vinegar.
✓   Garlic.
✓   Fresh basil.
✓   Truffles.
✓   Butter.

The healthiest types of food are vegetables, fruit, and whole grains. The least healthy types of food are red meat and processed foods. If those two categories are combined, processed foods are the least healthy. Processed cheeses, table salt, oils, sauces, dressings, and condiments are the worst of the worst.

The cold-pressed extra virgin olive oil is incredible. It's delicious drizzled on just about anything, and it is a healthy fat that helps lower the risk of heart disease and can reduce the risk of stroke and help lower cancer risk.

You don't need to "eat the Mediterranean diet". You just need the Mediterranean diet. Healthy vegetables, fruits, nuts, cheese, and whole grains.

Why the Mediterranean Diet?

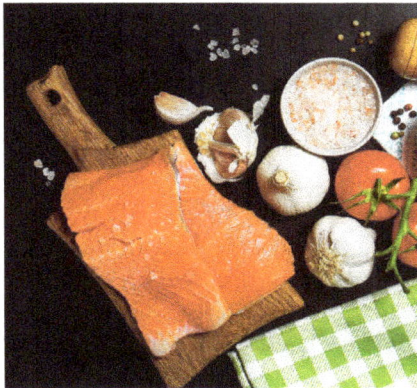

The Mediterranean diet gained popularity in the medical fields because of its documented benefits to heart health. But, plenty of research has shown that the Mediterranean diet can have a much longer list of health benefits that go beyond the heart. This chapter will go over just a few of the many improvements you can experience with your health when you start on the Mediterranean diet.

Heart Health and Reduced Risk of Stroke

The Mediterranean diet first gained attention because of the significantly low numbers of reported coronary heart disease in the regions of the Mediterranean. There are many components of the Mediterranean diet that help promote heart health. By reducing and eventually eliminating your consumption of processed foods, refined grains, and processed meats you reduce your risk of a number of heart conditions including heart attack and stroke. The diet focuses on replacing unhealthy trans fats with healthier unsaturated or monounsaturated fats. Fresh fish, fruits, and vegetables that are high in fiber, omega-3 fatty acids, and antioxidants are consumed daily.

Heart health is greatly impacted by diet. Maintaining healthy levels of good cholesterol, blood pressure, blood sugar, and staying within a healthy weight results in optimal heart health.

Your diet directly affects each of these components.

Those who are at greater risk are often advised to begin adhering to a low-fat diet. A low-fat diet cuts out all fats including those from oils, nuts, and red meats. Studies have shown that the Mediterranean diet, which includes healthy fats, is more effective at lowering cardiovascular risks than a standard low-fat diet (Are processed red meats, 2019). This is because the unsaturated fats consumed on the Mediterranean diet not only lower bad cholesterol levels, but also increase good cholesterol levels.

The Mediterranean diet also stresses the importance of daily activity and stress reduction by enjoying quality time with friends and family. Each of these elements, along with eating more plant-based foods, significantly improves heart health and reduces the risk of many heart-related conditions. By increasing your intake of fresh fruits and vegetables while adding in regular daily activities, you improve not just your heart health but overall health.

Reduces Age-Related Muscle and Bone Weakness

Eating a well-balanced diet that provides you with a wide range of vitamins and minerals is essential for reducing muscle weakness and bone degradation. This is especially important as you age. Accident-related injuries such as tripping, falling or slipping while walking can cause serious injury. As you age, this becomes even more of a concern as some simple falls can be fatal. Many accidents occur because of weakening muscle mass and the loss of bone density. Women, especially those who are entering the menopause phase of their life, are at a greater risk of serious injury from accidental falls because the estrogen levels decline significantly at this time. This decrease in estrogen results in a loss of bone and muscle mass. The decrease of estrogen can also cause bone-thinning which over time develops into osteoporosis.

Maintaining healthy bone mass and muscle agility as you age can be challenging. When you are not getting the proper nutrients to promote healthy bones and muscles, you increase your risk of developing osteoporosis. The Mediterranean diet offers you a simple way to fulfill the dietary needs necessary to improve bone and muscle functioning.

Antioxidants, vitamins C and K, carotenoids, magnesium, potassium, and phytoestrogens are essential minerals and nutrients for optimal musculoskeletal health. Plant-based foods, unsaturated fats, and whole grains help provide you with the necessary balance of nutrients that keep your bones and muscles healthy. Sticking with a Mediterranean diet can improve and reduce the loss of bone mass as you age.

Reduces the Risk of Alzheimer's

Alzheimer's disease is a form of dementia where there is significant cognitive decline. Those with Alzheimer's suffer from:

- Disorientation
- Memory loss
- Inability to think clearly
- Speech problems
- Impaired judgment
- Visual and spatial disorientation

Alzheimer's is a common brain disorder in older adults, 60 years of age or older, but the first signs of Alzheimer's can be present in adults as young as 30 years of age. The condition can progress fast or slowly depending on how quickly the neurons in the brain begin to die off. Though the decline begins in the hippocampus area of the brain it becomes widespread as it progresses.

Individuals with Alzheimer's show a significant increase in beta-amyloid proteins in the brain and have a much lower level of brain energy. Research has focused on trying to identify those who are at greater risk of dementia early on through brain scans and imaging. In one such study, brain scans were conducted on 70 individuals between the ages of 30 and 60. None of the participants showed signs of dementia and 34 of them adhered to a Mediterranean diet while 36 followed a standard Western diet. When brain scans were conducted at the beginning of the study and then two years later. The scans showed that those on the Western diet had significant loss in brain energy levels and an increase in the beta-amyloid build-up as opposed to those on the Mediterranean diet (Mediterranean Diet May Slow Development, 2018). The study highlights how simple lifestyle changes, such as those suggested on the Mediterranean diet, can help reduce the risk of Alzheimer's and other cognitive declines.

This indicates that diet can have an impact on the leading two signifiers of the development of Alzheimer's disease. Just as diet can impact other areas of your health, it can affect your brain health as well. Cholesterol, blood sugar, and blood vessel health can contribute to your risk of developing Alzheimer's disease. The most common sources of fuel for the brain are fresh fruits vegetables that supply it with vital vitamins and nutrients. When processed foods, refined grains, and added sugars are consumed too often, this impairs the brain's functionality as these foods release toxins into the body. These toxins then cause widespread inflammation and the brain begins to build up plaque which causes a malfunction of cognitive ability (Nutrition and Dementia, 2019).

The Western diet consists of a number of foods that increase the risk of Alzheimer's disease such as processed meat, refined grains like white bread and pasta, and added sugar. Foods that contain diacetyl, which is a chemical commonly used in the refinement process, increase beta-amyloid plaque build-up in the brain. Microwaveable popcorn, margarine, and butter are some of the most consumed foods that contain this harmful chemical. It is no wonder that Alzheimer's is becoming one of the leading causes of death among Americans.

The Mediterranean diet, on the other hand, includes a wide range of foods that have been proven to boost memory and slow down cognitive decline. Dark leafy vegetables, fresh berries, extra virgin olive oil, and fresh fish contain brain-boosting vitamins and minerals that can improve brain health. The Mediterranean diet can help you make the necessary diet and lifestyle changes that can greatly decrease your risk of Alzheimer's.

Reduces Risk of Parkinson's Disease

Parkinson's disease is a slowly progressing neurodegenerative illness that distresses the dopamine-producing neurons in the brain. Those with Parkinson's disease will suffer from:

- Tremors
- Muscle stiffness
- Balance troubles
- Difficulty walking
- Depression
- Sleep problems
- Cognitive disruptions

There is no cure for Parkinson's and medications and therapies suggested for this condition only helps individuals manage symptoms, not slow or stop the progress of the disease. Genetics and environmental factors have been researched to better understand what causes one to develop Parkinson's disease. While genetics plays a factor in exposure to pesticides, herbicides, high cholesterol, low vitamin D levels, and limited physical activity can all increase the risk of Parkinson's disease.

Parkinson's disease is also common among individuals who have a higher level of oxidative stress. This damages the cells in the brain and can result in serious cognitive and physical decline. Antioxidants can help reduce the risk of developing Parkinson's disease and can help repair damaged cells and form stronger connections in the brain.

The Mediterranean diet encourages the consumption of antioxidant-rich foods such as fresh fruits and vegetables. Eating organic and locally grown fruits and vegetables reduces the risk of toxin exposure from pesticides and herbicides.

Those with Parkinson's are often encouraged to change their diet so that it includes more healthy fats, like extra virgin olive oil, seeds, and nuts, fresh fruits, organic vegetables, and whole grains. This diet recommendation is the basis of the Mediterranean diet. Individuals are also encouraged to reduce the consumption of salt, sugar, and empty calorie foods. Which is also what the Mediterranean diet encourages.

Protects Against Type 2 Diabetes

The Mediterranean diet is the most recommended diet from health professionals for those diagnosed with Type 2 diabetes or prediabetes. The combination of healthy foods and regular exercise that the Mediterranean diet promotes are two of the key components to help individuals manage and even see a remission of symptoms.

Type 2 diabetes develops when your body is no longer able to produce or use the insulin produced properly. This causes blood sugar levels to spike to dangerous levels. Your blood sugar or glucose is what gives your body energy. It supplies fuel to your muscles, tissues, and cells so they are able to function properly. When glucose is released into the bloodstream it signals the pancreas to begin to produce insulin so that the cells in the body can properly absorb the glucose. When you have type 2 diabetes your pancreas is either not making enough insulin, and therefore your cells are not able to absorb enough of it, or the insulin is not being used properly so glucose is remaining in the body. A build-up of glucose in your body can cause a long list of health complications. The body may turn to use its own muscle and fat to get the energy it needs. Blood vessels can also become damaged which increases the risk of heart attack and stroke.

Those who are at the greatest risk of developing Type 2 diabetes include:

- Individuals who are overweight or obese
- Individuals who have limited physical activity.
- Individuals who have a family history of Type 2 diabetes
- Individuals who have insulin resistance

The most common symptoms of Type 2 diabetes include

- Excessive fatigue
- Frequent numbness of the hands or feet
- Tingling feelings in the hands and feet
- Regular headaches
- Vision difficulties
- Increase in urination
- Unquenchable thirst

How to Start

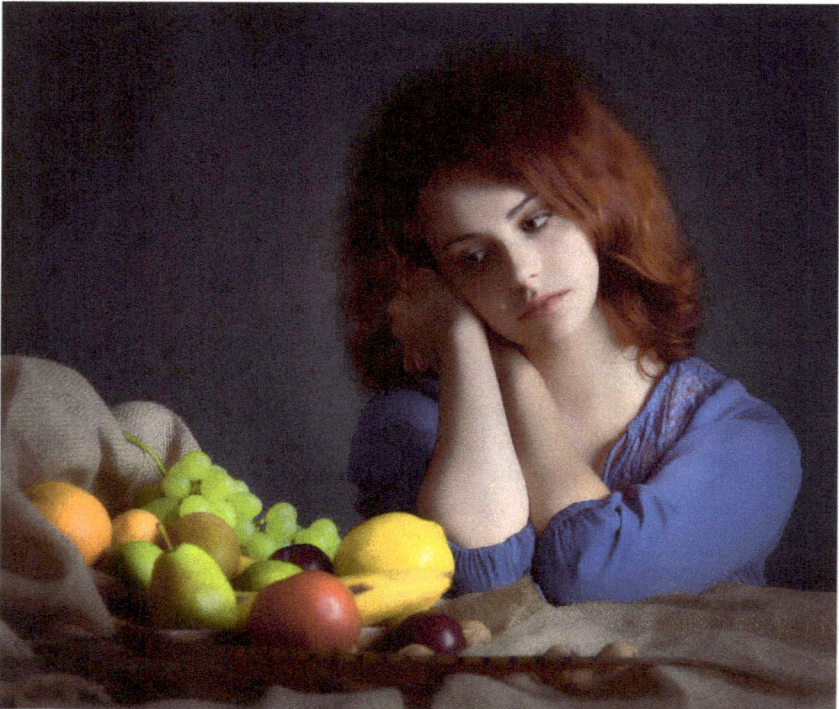

It's important that you have the right ingredients on hand, know about some of the foods you'll be eating, and have an idea of the meals you'd like to prepare. You'll also want to gradually (or immediately, if you're really eager) rid the house of the foods that you'll no longer be eating.

While there are no supplements or specially packaged foods to buy, there are several key ingredients that you'll need to stock up on, and you'll also want to locate sources for the freshest and most healthful fruits, vegetables, and fish.

Preparing for the Mediterranean diet is largely about preparing yourself for a new way of eating, adjusting your attitude toward food into one of joyful expectation and appreciation of good meals and good company. It's as much a mindset as anything else, so you'll want to make your environment one in which the Mediterranean way of eating can be naturally followed and easily enjoyed.

Preparing for the Mediterranean diet can be as simple as getting out the good dishes so that you can fully enjoy your meals or visiting a few local markets to check out the freshness and prices of their offerings.

You can take a month to prepare your pantry and yourself, or you can take just a few days, but a little time spent in advance can make all the difference in those first few weeks of your healthful new lifestyle.

Planning Your Mediterranean Diet

With the Mediterranean diet, you don't need to run out and buy special appliances, hard-to-find or expensive ingredients, special supplements, or even new workout gear, but there are a few things that will make your transition to the diet easier and more fun.

Ease Your Way into More Healthful Eating

Before actually starting the diet, it can be helpful to spend a week or two cutting back on the least healthful foods that you currently eat. You might start with fast food if you frequent the drive-through, or eliminate cream-based sauces and soups. You can then start cutting back on processed foods like chips, boxed dinners, and frozen meals.

Some other things to start trimming might be sodas, coffee with a lot of milk and sugar, butter, and red meats such as beef, pork, and lamb. You don't have to eliminate these things entirely during this period, but you'd be surprised at how quickly your body adjusts if you gradually wean yourself from them. This can make it much easier to adapt to the diet once you do begin in earnest.

Start Thinking About What You'll Be Eating

When you're planning a vacation, you spend a lot of time looking through brochures, scanning websites, and reading books about your destination. It builds anticipation, informs you, and helps you make the best choices once you arrive. It's all part of the fun of traveling somewhere wonderful and new.

Gather What You'll Need

Everything in the Mediterranean diet is easily found at grocery stores, farmers' markets, and seafood shops.

Find out where your local farmers' markets are and spend a leisurely morning checking out what's available. Whenever possible, you'll want to buy seasonal fruits and vegetables, so talk to farmers about what they harvest and when. Small farmers love to talk about what they do and why they're so passionate about the food they grow. Building relationships with those vendors can lead not only to great new friendships, but also to getting special deals and the best selection, finding out ahead of time what's coming to market, and often some great recipes, too.

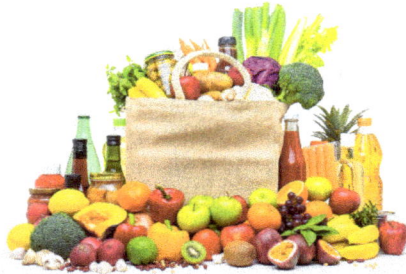

The Top Ten Tips for Success

Here are the best ways, some large and some small, to help ensure that you enjoy your Mediterranean diet to the fullest. These strategies can also help you lose weight, if that's one of your goals, by making it easier for you to adjust to the diet and stick with it.

1. *Treat Yourself Like Company*
2. *The Mediterranean diet is as much about how you eat as it is about what you eat. The Mediterranean people have a respect for and appreciation of food that inspires them to set beautiful (though often very simple) tables. Bring out the good china, put some fresh flowers in a canning jar, light some candles, or eat outside on the patio. However, you choose to do it, treat every meal as though you were having guests.*

1. *Learn to Savor*
2. *In our fast-paced multitasking culture, we have a tendency to eat without paying attention to our food. We eat standing up or while driving to work,*

watching TV, or finishing up some paperwork. This is the antithesis of Mediterranean custom, where it's not uncommon to linger over even a simple meal for a couple of hours and where the idea of doing anything mundane while eating just seems silly.

3. *Turn off the TV, even if you're eating alone. Put away the work, the cell phone, and any other distractions. Even if you're having dinner for one, focus on the delicious food you're eating. Really taste what's on your plate and start appreciating the pleasure of flavor.*

1. *Become a Social Eater*
2. *Gathering around food is something that families and friends do every day in the Mediterranean, even if all that's being served is some crusty bread with good olive oil. While Sunday afternoon dinners are traditionally an important part of the week in the Mediterranean region, even simple meals are an excuse to invite someone over for good food and conversation. Even when there are no guests, families will linger at the table to talk about the day and enjoy each other's presence.*
3. *Inviting friends and family over for a simple summer lunch or a casual dinner party is a great way to incorporate the Mediterranean approach to dining into your own life. For the Mediterranean people, eating is as much about the company as it is about the food, and meals really do taste better when you share them.*

1. *Learn to Make Substitutions*
2. *Very few things are off-limits in the Mediterranean diet, but moderation is key. You may find that the thing that stands in for your favorite junk food becomes your new favorite!*
3. *Kale chips taste better than commercial potato chips and they can be made without all of the unhealthful fat, excess salt, and preservatives. A refreshing homemade granita takes no time to make, the flavor is unparalleled, and it's much better for you than that ice cream you're used to.*

1. *Get Some Moderate Exercise Every Day—Preferably Outdoors*
2. *In the Mediterranean region, spending time outdoors is just a natural part of any day. Sunshine and good weather abound in the area, as do beautiful scenery and warm oceans. People spend as much time outside as they do inside, whether they're working in the garden, walking on the beach, or throwing a ball for the dog.*
3. *Try to get at least thirty minutes of moderate exercise three times per week. This has been shown to be an important element of losing weight, improving cardiovascular health, and attaining an overall feeling of happiness and well-being.*

4. *Try walking in the morning or after work, taking a ballroom dancing class, swimming in the pool or ocean, playing a game of catch with the kids, or any other activity that gets you moving. It doesn't have to be strenuous and it doesn't have to be the same activity every day—in fact, it shouldn't be.*

1. *Don't Tempt Yourself*
2. *Don't keep pastries in the pantry for visiting neighbors or chicken nuggets in the freezer just because they haven't expired yet. Having foods at home that are not part of the diet or that you tend to overindulge in is just tempting fate. If you need something to serve guests, the Mediterranean menu offers plenty of choices. There is no occasion for which you will need chicken nuggets. Give them to the family next door!*

1. *Don't Overwhelm Yourself*
2. *Try not to complicate your life by preparing three weeks' worth of menus at the get-go or trying ten new recipes in a week. Take things slowly, and cultivate a relaxed approach to your new way of eating. Try a few new recipes, but make sure they're not all complicated dishes that'll just stress you out. Most Mediterranean dishes are simple, with few ingredients and very straightforward preparation. You don't need a lot of fancy steps to make great meals.*

1. *Give Yourself a Break*
2. *So you snuck out to the fast-food place and ate the messiest and most calorie-laden burger they sell. Hopefully it was truly yummy. Now move on.*
3. *One slip up won't kill you. Do not spend three days eating garbage because you're upset about that slipup!*

1. *Try Something New Each Week*
2. *Eating the Mediterranean way should be fun, exciting, and even a little exotic. Try to choose one unfamiliar fruit, vegetable, fish, or another ingredient each week. It'll keep things interesting and enhance that sense of voyaging to another land.*

1. *Try Growing Your Own*
2. *The people of the Mediterranean region are very garden-focused. It's common for them to have lush kitchen gardens in their backyards, and even many city dwellers insist on a few pots of fresh herbs on the windowsill. Growing your own herbs and vegetables is fun, saves money, and is the best way to taste something at its very freshest.*

1

Breakfast

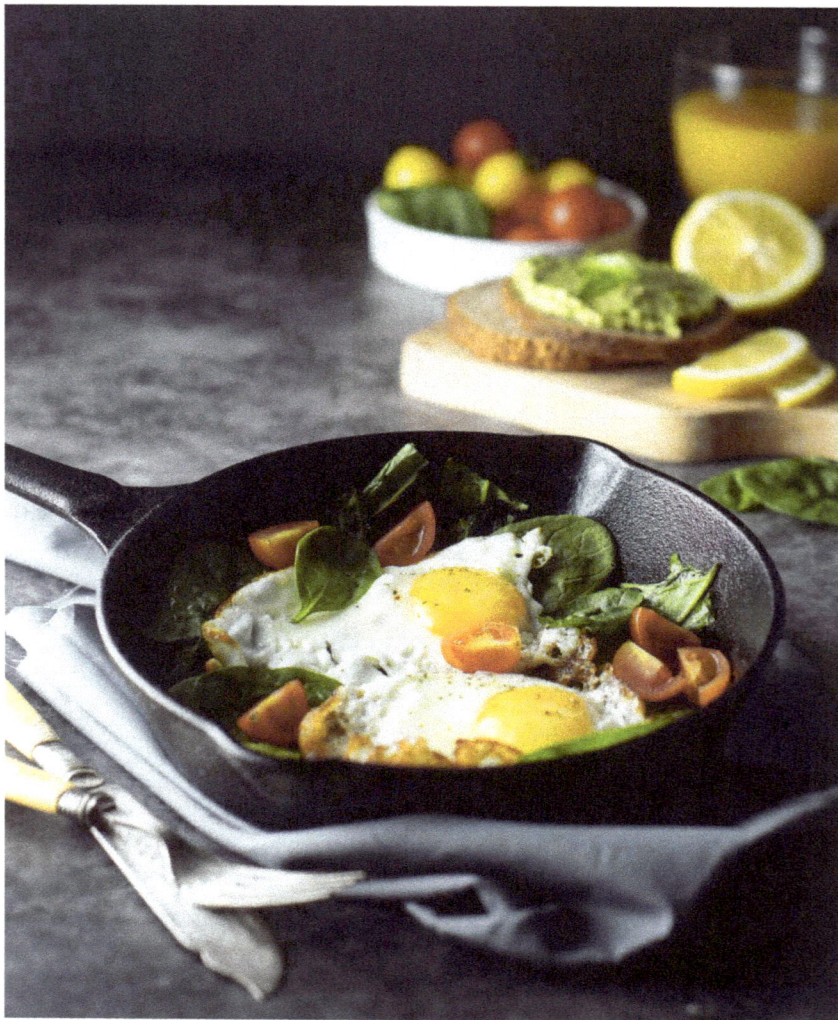

Mediterranean Breakfast Salad

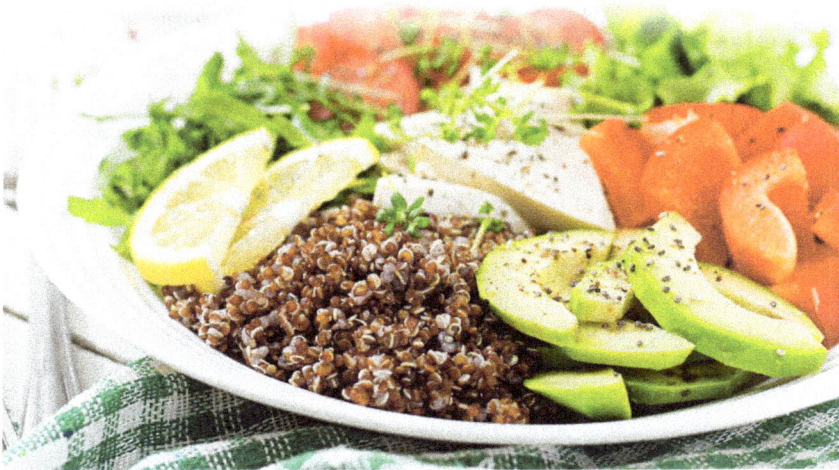

Preparation Time: 10 Minutes
Cooking Time: 20 Minutes
Servings: 4
Nutrition:
Calories: 85
Protein: 3.4 g
Fat: 3.46 g
Carbs: 6.71 g

Ingredients:

- 4 whole eggs
- 2 cups of cherry tomatoes or heirloom tomatoes cut in half or wedges
- 10 cups of arugula
- A 1/2 chopped seedless cucumber
- 1 large avocado
- 1 cup cooked or cooled quinoa
- 1/2 cup of chopped mixed herbs like dill and mint
- 1 cup of chopped Almonds
- 1 lemon
- extra virgin olive oil

- sea salt
- freshly ground black pepper

Directions:

1. In this recipe, the eggs are the first thing that needs to be cooked. Start with soft boiling the eggs. To do that, you need to get water in a pan and let it sit to boil. Once it starts boiling, reduces the heat to simmer and lower the eggs into the water and let them cook for about 6 minutes. After they are boiled, wash the eggs with cold water and set aside. Peel them when they are cool and ready to use.
2. Combine quinoa, arugula, cucumbers, and tomatoes in a bowl and add a little bit of olive oil over the top. Toss it with salt and pepper to equally season all of it.
3. Once all that is done, serve the salad on four plates and garnish it with sliced avocados and the halved eggs. After that, season it with some more pepper and salt.
4. To top it all off, then use almonds and sprinkle some herbs along with some lemon zest and olive oil.

Smoked Salmon and Poached Eggs on Toast

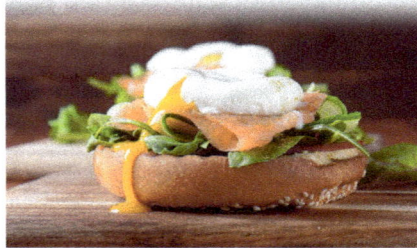

Preparation Time: 10 Minutes
Cooking Time: 4 Minutes
Servings: 4

Nutrition:
Calories: 459
Protein: 31 g
Fat: 22 g

Carbs: 33 g

Ingredients:

- 2 oz avocado smashed
- 2 slices of bread toasted
- Pinch of kosher salt and cracked black pepper
- 1/4 tsp freshly squeezed lemon juice
- 2 eggs see notes, poached
- 3.5 oz smoked salmon
- 1 TBSP. thinly sliced scallions
- Splash of Kikkoman soy sauce optional
- Microgreens are optional

Directions:

1. Take a small bowl and then smash the avocado into it. Then, add the lemon juice and also a pinch of salt into the mixture. Then, mix it well and set aside.
2. After that, poach the eggs and toast the bread for some time.
3. Once the bread is toasted, you will have to spread the avocado on both slices and after that, add the smoked salmon to each slice.
4. Thereafter, carefully transfer the poached eggs to the respective toasts.
5. Add a splash of Kikkoman soy sauce and some cracked pepper; then, just garnish with scallions and microgreens.

Honey Almond Ricotta Spread with Peaches

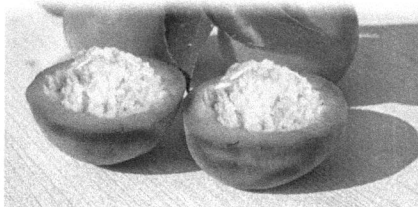

Preparation Time: 5 Minutes
Cooking Time: 8 Minutes
Servings: 4

. . .

Nutrition:
Calories: 187
Protein: 7 g
Fat: 9 g
Carbs: 18 g

Ingredients:

- 1/2 cup Fisher Sliced Almonds
- 1 cup whole milk ricotta
- 1/4 teaspoon almond extract
- zest from an orange, optional
- 1 teaspoon honey
- hearty whole-grain toast
- English muffin or bagel
- extra Fisher sliced almonds
- sliced peaches
- extra honey for drizzling

Directions:

1. Cut peaches into a proper shape and then brush them with olive oil. After that, set it aside.
2. Take a bowl; combine the ingredients for the filling. Set aside.
3. Then just pre-heat grill to medium.
4. Place peaches cut side down onto the greased grill.
5. Close lid cover and then just grill until the peaches have softened, approximately 6-10 minutes, depending on the size of the peaches.
6. Then you will have to place peach halves onto a serving plate.
7. Put a spoon of about 1 tablespoon of ricotta mixture into the cavity (you are also allowed to use a small scooper).
8. Sprinkle it with slivered almonds, crushed amaretti cookies, and honey.

Mediterranean Eggs Cups

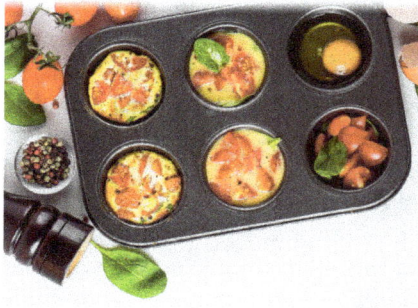

Preparation Time: 10 Minutes
Cooking Time: 20 Minutes
Servings: 8
Nutrition:
Calories: 240
Protein: 9 g
Fat: 16 g
Carbs: 13 g

Ingredients:

- 1 dough sheet
- 1 cup spinach, finely diced
- 1/2 yellow onion, finely diced
- 1/2 cup sliced sun-dried tomatoes
- 4 large basil leaves, finely diced
- Pepper and salt to taste
- 1/3 cup feta cheese crumbles
- 8 large eggs
- 1/4 cup milk (any kind)

Directions:

1. You have to heat the oven to 375°F.
2. Then, roll the dough sheet into a 12x8-inch rectangle
3. Then, cut in half lengthwise
4. After that, you will have to cut each half crosswise into 4 pieces, forming 8 (4x3-inch) pieces dough. Then, press each into the bottom and up sides of the ungreased muffin cup.

5. Trim dough to keep the dough from touching, if essential. Set aside.
6. Then, you will have to combine the eggs, salt, pepper in the bowl and beat it with a whisk until well mixed. Set aside.
7. Melt the butter in 12-inch skillet over medium heat until sizzling; add bell peppers.
8. You will have to cook it, stirring occasionally, 2-3 minutes or until crisply tender.
9. After that, add spinach leaves; continue cooking until spinach is wilted. Then just add egg mixture and prosciutto.
10. Divide the mixture evenly among prepared muffin cups.
11. Finally, bake it for 14-17 minutes or until the crust is golden brown.

Low-Carb Baked Eggs with Avocado and Feta

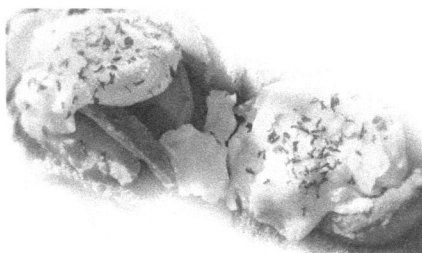

Preparation Time: 10 Minutes
Cooking Time: 15 Minutes
Servings: 2

Nutrition:
Calories: 280
Protein: 11 g
Fat: 23 g
Carbs: 10 g

Ingredients:

- 1 avocado
- 4 eggs

- 2-3 tbsp. crumbled feta cheese
- Nonstick cooking spray
- Pepper and salt to taste

Directions:

1. First, you will have to preheat the oven to 400 degrees F.
2. After that, when the oven is on the proper temperature, you will have to put the gratin dishes right on the baking sheet.
3. Then, leave the dishes to heat in the oven for almost 10 minutes
4. After that process, you need to break the eggs into individual ramekins.
5. Then, let the avocado and eggs come to room temperature for at least 10 minutes
6. Then, peel the avocado properly and cut it each half into 6-8 slices
7. You will have to remove the dishes from the oven and spray them with the non-stick spray
8. Then, you will have to arrange all the sliced avocados in the dishes and tip two eggs into each dish
9. Sprinkle with feta, add pepper and salt to taste

Mediterranean Eggs White Breakfast Sandwich with Roasted Tomatoes

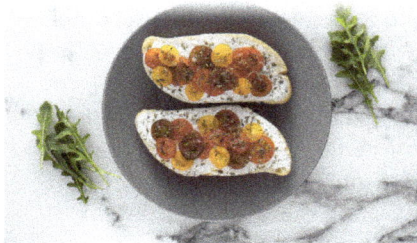

Preparation Time: 15 Minutes
Cooking Time: 10 Minutes
Servings: 2
Nutrition:
Calories: 458
Protein: 21 g
Fat: 24 g

Carbs: 51 g

Ingredients:

- Salt and pepper to taste
- ¼ cup egg whites
- 1 teaspoon chopped fresh herbs like rosemary, basil, parsley,
- 1 whole-grain seeded ciabatta roll
- 1 teaspoon butter
- 1-2 slices Muenster cheese
- 1 tablespoon pesto
- About ½ cup roasted tomatoes
- 10 ounces grape tomatoes
- 1 tablespoon extra-virgin olive oil
- Black pepper and salt to taste

Directions:

1. First, you will have to melt the butter over medium heat in the small nonstick skillet.
2. Then, mix the egg whites with pepper and salt.
3. Then, sprinkle it with the fresh herbs
4. After that cook it for almost 3-4 minutes or until the eggs are done, then flip it carefully
5. Meanwhile, toast ciabatta bread in the toaster
6. After that, you will have to place the egg on the bottom half of the sandwich rolls, then top with cheese
7. Add roasted tomatoes and the top half of roll.
8. To make a roasted tomato, preheat the oven to 400 degrees.
9. Then, slice the tomatoes in half lengthwise.
10. Place on the baking sheet and drizzle with olive oil.
11. Season it with pepper and salt and then roast in the oven for about 20 minutes. Skins will appear wrinkled when done.

Greek Yogurt Pancakes

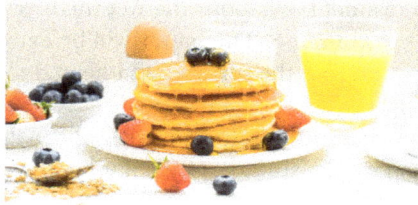

Preparation Time: 10 Minutes
Cooking Time: 5 Minutes
Servings: 2

Nutrition:
Calories: 166
Protein: 14 g
Fat: 5 g
Carbs: 52g

Ingredients:

- 1 cup all-purpose flour
- 1 cup whole-wheat flour
- 1/4 teaspoon salt
- 4 teaspoons baking powder
- 1 Tablespoon sugar
- 1 1/2 cups unsweetened almond milk
- 2 teaspoons vanilla extract
- 2 large eggs
- 1/2 cup plain 2% Greek yogurt
- Fruit, for serving
- Maple syrup, for serving

Directions:

1. First, you will have to pour the curds into the bowl and mix them well until creamy.
2. You will have to put egg whites then mix them well until combined.

3. Then take a distinct bowl, pour the wet mixture into the dry mixture. Stir to combine. The batter will be extremely thick.
4. Spoon the batter onto the sprayed pan heated to medium-high.
5. Then, you will have to flip the pancakes once when they begin to bubble a bit on the surface. Cook until golden brown on both sides.

Mediterranean Feta and Quinoa Egg Muffins

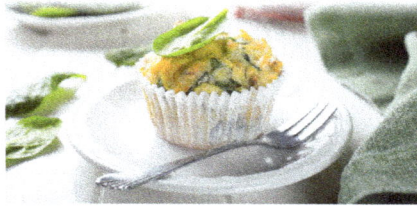

Preparation Time: 15 Minutes
Cooking Time: 15 Minutes
Servings: 12

Nutrition:
Calories: 113
Protein: 6 g
Fat: 7 g
Carbs: 5 g
Ingredients:

- 2 cups baby spinach finely chopped
- 1 cup chopped or sliced cherry tomatoes
- 1/2 cup finely chopped onion
- 1 tablespoon chopped fresh oregano
- 1 cup crumbled feta cheese
- 1/2 cup chopped {pitted} kalamata olives
- 2 teaspoons high oleic sunflower oil
- 1 cup cooked quinoa
- 8 eggs

- 1/4 teaspoon salt

Directions:

1. Pre-heat oven to 350 degrees Fahrenheit
2. Make 12 silicone muffin holders on the baking sheet, or just grease a 12-cup muffin tin with oil and set aside.
3. Finely slice the vegetables
4. Heat the skillet to medium.
5. Add the vegetable oil and onions and sauté for 2 minutes.
6. Then, add tomatoes and sauté for another minute, then add spinach and sauté until wilted, about 1 minute.
7. Put the beaten egg into a bowl and then add lots of vegetables like feta cheese, quinoa, veggie mixture as well as salt, and then stir well until everything is properly combined.
8. Pour the ready mixture into greased muffin tins or silicone cups, dividing the mixture equally. Then, bake it in an oven for 30 minutes or so, or until the eggs set nicely, and the muffins turn a light golden brown in color.

Mediterranean Eggs

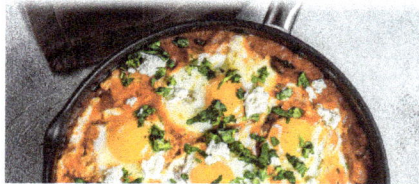

Preparation Time: 15 Minutes
Cooking Time: 20 Minutes
Servings: 2

Nutrition:
Calories: 304
Protein: 12 g
Fat: 16 g
Carbs: 28 g

. . .

Ingredients:

- 5 tbsp. of divided olive oil
- 2 diced medium-sized Spanish onions
- 2 diced red bell peppers
- 2 minced cloves garlic
- 1 teaspoon cumin seeds
- 4 diced large ripe tomatoes
- 1 tablespoon of honey
- Salt
- Freshly ground black pepper
- 1/3 cup crumbled feta
- 4 eggs
- 1 teaspoon zaatar spice
- Grilled pita during serving

Directions:

1. To start with, you have to add 3 tablespoons of olive oil into a pan and heat it over medium heat. Along with the oil, sauté the cumin seeds, onions, garlic, and red pepper for a few minutes.
2. After that, add the diced tomatoes and salt and pepper to taste and cook them for about 10 minutes till they come together and form a light sauce.
3. With that, half the preparation is already done. Now you just have to break the eggs directly into the sauce and poach them. However, you must keep in mind to cook the egg whites but keep the yolks still runny. This takes about 8 to 10 minutes.
4. While plating adds some feta and olive oil with zaatar spice to further enhance the flavors. Once done, serve with grilled pita.

Pastry-Less Spanakopita

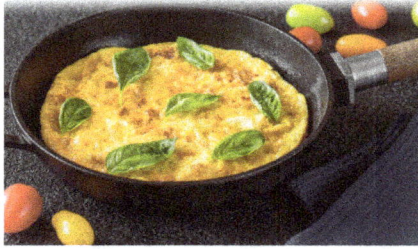

Preparation Time: 5 Minutes
Cooking Time: 20 Minutes
Servings: 4

Nutrition:

Calories: 325
Protein: 11.2 g
Fat: 27.9 g
Carbs: 7.3 g

Ingredients:

- 1/8 teaspoons black pepper, add as per taste
- 1/3 cup of virgin olive oil
- 4 lightly beaten eggs
- 7 cups of Lettuce, preferably a spring mix (mesclun)
- 1/2 cup of crumbled Feta cheese
- 1/8 teaspoon of Sea salt, add to taste
- 1 finely chopped medium Yellow onion

Directions:

1. For this delicious recipe, you need to first start by preheating the oven to 180C and grease the flan dish.
2. Once done, pour the extra virgin olive oil into a large saucepan and heat it over medium heat with the onions, until they are translucent. To that, add greens and keep stirring until all the ingredients are wilted.
3. After completing that, you should season it with salt and pepper

and transfer the greens to the prepared dish and sprinkle on some feta cheese.

4. Pour the eggs and bake it for 20 minutes till it is cooked through and slightly brown.

Date and Walnut Overnight Oats

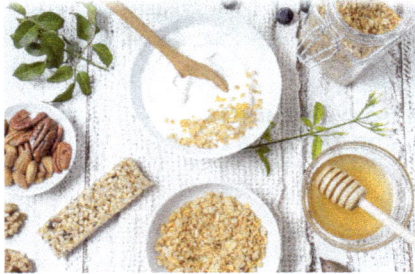

Preparation Time: 5 Minutes
Cooking Time: 20 Minutes
Servings: 2

Nutrition:
Calories: 350
Protein: 14 g
Fat: 12 g
Carbs: 49 g
Ingredients:

- ¼ Cup Greek Yogurt, Plain
- 1/3 cup of yogurt
- 2/3 cup of oats
- 1 cup of milk
- 2 tsp date syrup or you can also use maple syrup or honey
- 1 mashed banana
- ¼ tsp cinnamon
- ¼ cup walnuts
- pinch of salt (approx.1/8 tsp)

Directions:

1. Firstly, get a mason jar or a small bowl and add all the ingredients.
2. After that stir and mix all the ingredients well.
3. Cover it securely, and cool it in a refrigerator overnight.
4. After that, take it out the next morning, add more liquid or cinnamon if required, and serve cold. (However, you can also microwave it for people with a warmer palate.)

Greek Quinoa Breakfast Bowl

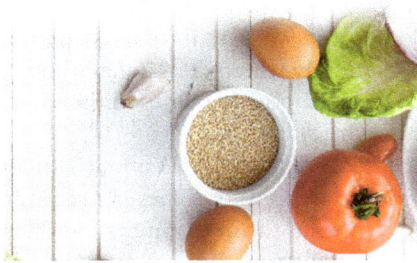

Preparation Time: 10 Minutes
Cooking Time: 20 Minutes
Servings: 2

Nutrition:
Calories: 357
Protein: 23 g
Fat: 20 g
Carbs: 20 g

Ingredients:

- 2 large eggs
- 3/4 cup Greek yogurt
- 2 cups of cooked quinoa
- 3/4 cup muhammara
- 3 ounces of baby spinach
- 4 ounces of marinated kalamata olives
- 6 ounces of sliced cherry tomatoes

- 1 halved lemon
- hot chili oil
- salt & pepper to taste
- fresh dill and sesame seeds to garnish

Directions:

1. Add all the ingredients, Greek yogurt, granulated garlic, onion powder, salt, and pepper, and whisk them all together and set aside.
2. In a different large saucepan, heat the olive oil on medium-high heat and add the spinach. You have to keep in mind to cook the spinach till it is slightly wilted. This takes about 3-4 minutes.
3. After that, cook the cherry tomatoes in the same skillet for 3-4 minutes till they are softened.
4. Stir in the egg mixture into this for about 7 to 9 minutes, until it has set and cooked them so that they get scrambled.
5. After the eggs have set, stir in the quinoa and feta and cook until it is heated all the way through and serve it hot with some fresh dill and sesame seeds to garnish.

Mediterranean Frittata

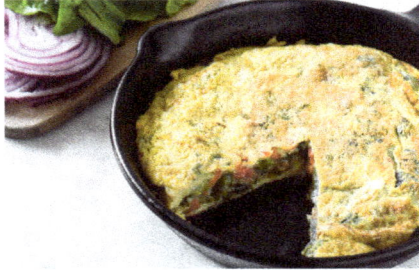

Preparation Time: 8 Minutes
Cooking Time: 6 Minutes
Servings: 4

Nutrition:
Calories: 178
Protein: 16 g
Fat: 12 g

Carbs: 2.2 g

Ingredients:

- Two teaspoons of olive oil
- 3/4 cup of baby spinach, packed
- Two green onions
- Four egg whites, large
- Six large eggs
- 1/3 cup of crumbled feta cheese, (1.3 ounces) along with sun-dried tomatoes and basil
- Two teaspoons of salt-free Greek seasoning
- 1/4 teaspoon of salt

Directions:

1. Take a boiler and preheat it
2. Take a ten-inch ovenproof skillet and pour the oil into it and keep the skillet on a medium flame.
3. While the oil gets heated, chop the spinach roughly and the onions.
4. Put the eggs, egg whites, Greek seasoning, cheese, as well as salt in a large mixing bowl and mix it thoroughly using a whisker.
5. Add the chopped spinach and onions into the mixing bowl and stir it well.
6. Pour the mixture into the pan and cook it for 2 minutes or more until the edges of the mixture set well. Lift the edges of the mixture gently and tilt the pan so that the uncooked portion can get underneath it. Cook for additional two minutes so that the whole mixture gets cooked properly.
7. Broil for two to three minutes till the center gets set.
8. Your Frittata is now ready. Serve it hot by cutting it into four wedges.

Honey-Caramelized Figs with Greek Yogurt

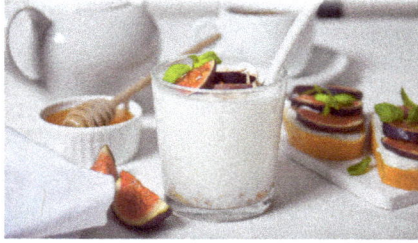

Preparation Time: 5 Minutes
Cooking Time: 5 Minutes
Servings: 4

Nutrition:

Calories: 350
Protein: 6 g
Fat: 19 g
Carbs: 40 g

Ingredients:

- Four fresh halved figs
- Two tablespoons of melted butter, 30ml
- Two tablespoons of brown sugar, 30ml
- Two cups of Greek yogurt 500ml
- 1/4 cup of honey, 60ml

Directions:

1. Take a non-stick skillet and preheat it over a medium flame
2. Put the butter on the pan and toss the figs into it and sprinkle in some brown sugar over it.
3. Put the figs on the pan and cut off the side of the figs.
4. Cook the figs on a medium flame for 2-3 minutes until they turn a golden brown.
5. Turn over the figs and cook them for 2-3 minutes again
6. Remove the figs from the pan and let it cool down a little.
7. Take a plate and put a scoop of Greek yogurt on it. Put the cooked figs over the yogurts and drizzle the honey over it

Savory Quinoa Egg Muffins with Spinach

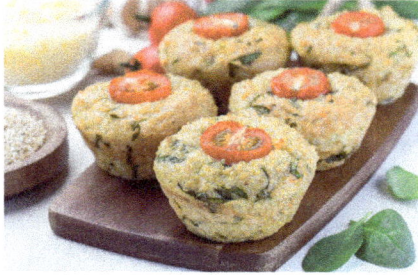

Preparation Time: 15 Minutes
Cooking Time: 20 Minutes
Servings: 2

Nutrition:
Calories: 61
Protein: 4 g
Fat: 3 g
Carbs: 6 g
Ingredients:

- One cup of quinoa
- Two cups of water/ vegetable broth)
- Four ounces of spinach which is about one cup
- Half chopped onion
- Two whole eggs
- 1/4 cup of grated cheese
- Half teaspoon of oregano or thyme
- Half teaspoon of garlic powder
- Half teaspoon of salt

Directions:

1. Take a medium saucepan and put water in it. Add the quinoa in the water and bring the whole thing to a simmer. Cover the pan and cook it for 10 minutes till the water gets absorbed by the quinoa. Remove the saucepan from the heat and let it cool down.

2. Take a nonstick pan and heat the onions till they turn soft and then add spinach. Cook all of them together till the spinach gets a little wilted and then remove it from the heat.
3. Preheat the oven to 176.667 C
4. Take a muffin pan and grease it lightly
5. Take a large bowl and add the cooked quinoa along with the cooked onions, spinach, and add cheese, eggs, thyme or oregano, salt, garlic powder, pepper and mix them together.
6. Put a spoonful of the mixture into a muffin tin. Make sure it is ¼ of a cup.
7. In the preheated pan, put it in the pan and bake it for around 20 minutes.

Avocado Tomato Gouda Socca Pizza

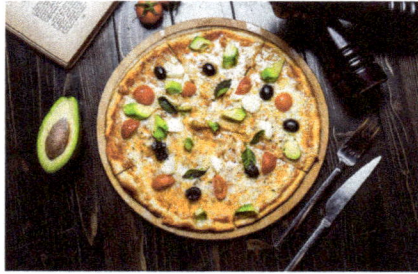

Preparation Time: 20 Minutes
Cooking Time: 20 Minutes
Servings: 2

Nutrition:
Calories: 416
Protein: 15 g
Fat: 10 g
Carbs: 37 g
Ingredients:

- One and 1/4 cups of chickpea or garbanzo bean flour
- One and 1/4 cups of cold water
- 1/4 teaspoon of pepper and sea salt each

- Two teaspoons of avocado or olive oil. Take one teaspoon extra for heating the pan
- One teaspoon of minced Garlic which will be around two cloves
- One teaspoon of Onion powder/other herb seasoning powder
- Ten to twelve-inch cast iron pan
- One sliced tomato
- Half avocado
- Two ounces of thinly sliced Gouda
- 1/4-1/3 cup of Tomato sauce
- Two or three teaspoons of chopped green scallion/onion
- Sprouted greens for green
- Extra pepper/salt for sprinkling on top of the pizza
- Red pepper flakes

Directions:

1. Mix the flour with two teaspoons of olive oil, herbs, water, and whisk it until a smooth mixture form. Keep it at room temperature for around 15-20 minutes to let the batter settle
2. In the meantime, preheat the oven and place the pan inside the oven and let it get heated for around 10 minutes
3. When the pan gets preheated, chop up the vegetables into fine slices
4. Remove the pan after ten minutes using oven mitts
5. Put one teaspoon of oil and swirl it all around to coat the pan
6. Pour the batter into the pan then slant the pan so that the batter spreads evenly throughout the pan.
7. Turn down the over to 425f and place back the pan for 5-8 minutes
8. Remove the pan from the oven and add the sliced avocado, tomato and on top of that, add the gouda slices and the onion slices
9. Put the pizza into the oven then wait till the cheese get melted or the sides of the bread gets crusty and brown
10. Remove the pizza from the pan and add the microgreens on top, along with the toppings.

Sunny-Side Up Baked Eggs with Swiss Chard, Feta, and Basil

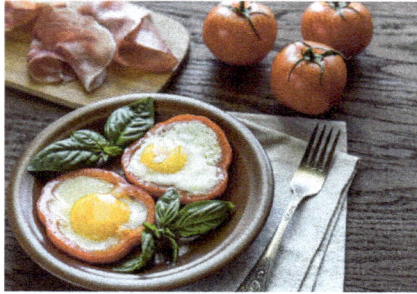

Preparation Time: 15 Minutes
Cooking Time: 10 Minutes
Servings: 4
Nutrition:
Calories: 270
Protein: 15 g
Fat: 19 g
Carbs: 12 g

Ingredients:

- 4 bell peppers, any color
- 1 tablespoon extra-virgin olive oil
- 8 large eggs
- ¾ teaspoon kosher salt, divided
- ¼ teaspoon freshly ground black pepper, divided
- 1 avocado, peeled, pitted, and diced
- ¼ cup red onion, diced
- ¼ cup fresh basil, chopped
- Juice of ½ lime

Directions:

1. Stem and seed the bell peppers. Cut 2 (2-inch-thick) rings from each pepper. Chop the remaining bell pepper into small dice and set aside.
2. Heat the olive oil in a large skillet over medium heat. Add 4 bell pepper rings, then crack 1 egg in the middle of each ring. Season with ¼ teaspoon of the salt and 1/8 teaspoon of the black pepper. Cook until the egg whites are generally set, but

the yolks are still runny 2 to 3 minutes. Gently flip and cook 1 additional minute for over easy. Move the egg–bell pepper rings to a platter or onto plates and repeats with the remaining 4 bell pepper rings.

3. In a medium bowl, blend the avocado, onion, basil, lime juice, reserved diced bell pepper, the remaining ¼ teaspoon kosher salt, and the remaining 1/8 teaspoon black pepper. Divide among the 4 plates.

Polenta with Sautéed Chard and Fried Eggs

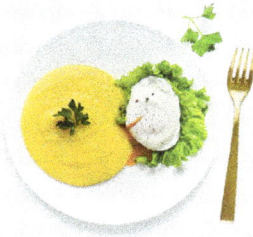

Preparation Time: 5 Minutes
Cooking Time: 20 Minutes
Servings: 4

Nutrition:
Calories: 310
Protein: 17 g
Fat: 18 g
Carbs: 21 g
Ingredients:

- 2½ cups water
- ½ teaspoon kosher salt
- ¾ cups whole-grain cornmeal
- ¼ teaspoon freshly ground black pepper
- 2 tablespoons grated Parmesan cheese
- 1 tablespoon extra-virgin olive oil
- 1 bunch (about 6 ounces) Swiss chard, leaves and stems chopped and separated

- 2 garlic cloves, sliced
- $1/4$ teaspoon kosher salt
- 1/8 teaspoon freshly ground black pepper
- Lemon juice (optional)
- 1 tablespoon extra-virgin olive oil
- 4 large eggs

Directions:
TO MAKE THE POLENTA

1. Le the water and salt to boil in a medium saucepan over high heat. Slowly add the cornmeal, whisking constantly.
2. Decrease the heat to low, cover, and cook for 10 to 15 minutes, stirring often to avoid lumps. Stir in the pepper and Parmesan and divide among 4 bowls.

TO MAKE THE CHARD

1. Heat the oil in a large frying pan on medium heat. Add the chard stems, garlic, salt, and pepper; sauté for 2 minutes. Add the chard leaves and cook until wilted, about 3 to 5 minutes.
2. Add a spritz of lemon juice (if desired), toss together, and divide evenly on top of the polenta.

TO MAKE THE EGGS

1. Heat the oil in the same large skillet over medium-high heat. Crack each egg into the skillet, taking care not to crowd the skillet and leaving space between the eggs. Cook until the whites are set and golden around the edges, about 2 to 3 minutes.
2. Serve sunny-side up or flip the eggs over carefully and cook 1 minute longer for over easy. Put one egg on top of the polenta and chard in each bowl.

Smoked Salmon Egg Scramble with Dill and Chives

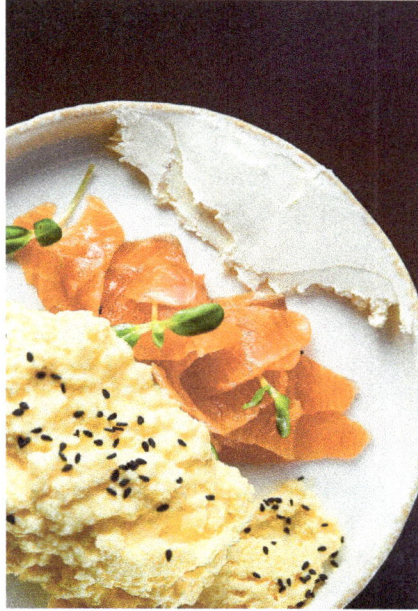

Preparation Time: 5 Minutes
Cooking Time: 5 Minutes
Servings: 2
Nutrition:
Calories: 325
Protein: 23 g
Fat: 26 g
Carbs: 1 g
Ingredients:

- 4 large eggs
- 1 tablespoon milk
- 1 tablespoon fresh chives, minced
- 1 tablespoon fresh dill, minced
- ¼ teaspoon kosher salt
- 1/8 teaspoon freshly ground black pepper
- 2 teaspoons extra-virgin olive oil
- 2 ounces smoked salmon, thinly sliced

Directions:

1. In a large bowl, blend together the eggs, milk, chives, dill, salt, and pepper.
2. Heat the olive oil in a medium skillet or sauté pan over medium heat. Add the egg mixture and cook for about 3 minutes, stirring occasionally.
3. Add the salmon and cook until the eggs are set but moist about 1 minute.

Eggs with Zucchini Noodles

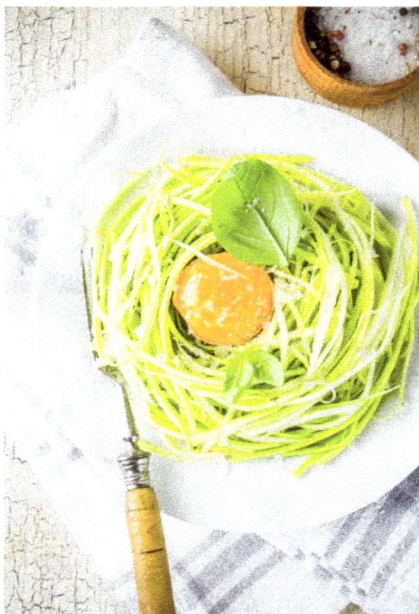

Preparation Time: 10 Minutes
Cooking Time: 11 Minutes
Servings: 2

Nutrition:
Calories: 296
Protein: 15 g
Fat: 24 g
Carbs: 11 g
Ingredients:

- 2 tablespoons extra-virgin olive oil
- 3 zucchinis, cut with a spiralizer
- 4 eggs
- Salt and black pepper to the taste
- A pinch of red pepper flakes
- Cooking spray
- 1 tablespoon basil, chopped

Directions:

1. In a bowl, combine the zucchini noodles with salt, pepper, and the olive oil, and toss well.
2. Grease a baking sheet with cooking spray and divide the zucchini noodles into 4 nests on it.
3. Crack an egg on top of each nest, sprinkle salt, pepper, and the pepper flakes on top, and bake at 350 degrees F for 11 minutes.
4. Divide the mix between plates, sprinkle the basil on top, and serve.

2

Snacks

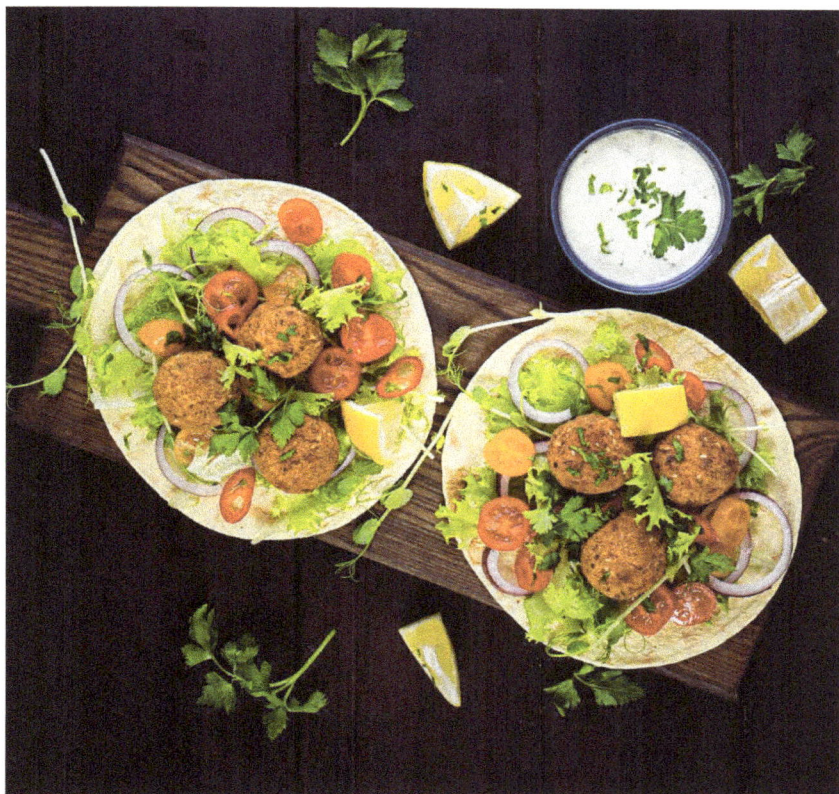

Meatballs Platter

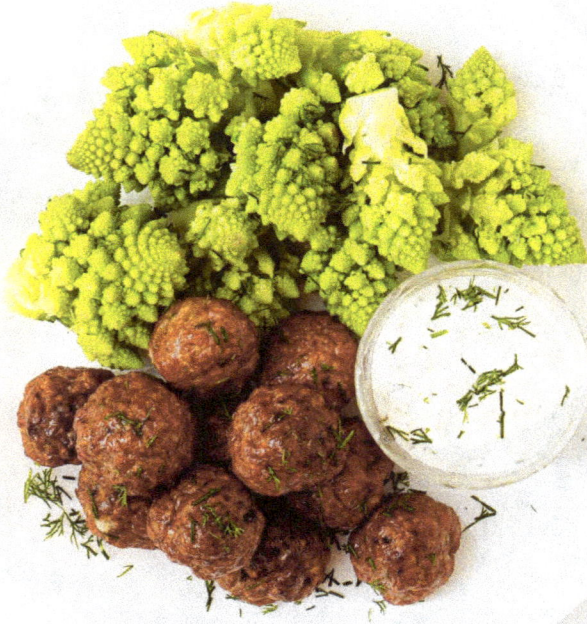

Preparation Time: 10 Minutes
Cooking Time: 15 Minutes
Servings: 4
Nutrition:
Calories: 300,
Fat: 15.4,
Fiber: 6.4,
Carbs: 22.4,
Protein: 35
Ingredients:

- 1-pound beef meat, ground
- ¼ cup panko breadcrumbs
- A pinch of salt and black pepper

- 3 tablespoons red onion, grated
- ¼ cup parsley, chopped
- 2 garlic cloves, minced
- 2 tablespoons lemon juice
- Zest of 1 lemon, grated
- 1 egg
- ½ teaspoon cumin, ground
- ½ teaspoon coriander, ground
- ¼ teaspoon cinnamon powder
- 2 ounces feta cheese, crumbled
- Cooking spray

Directions:

1. In a bowl, blend the beef with the breadcrumbs, salt, pepper and the rest of the ingredients except the cooking spray, stir well and shape medium balls out of this mix.
2. Arrange the meatballs on a baking sheet lined with parchment paper, grease them with cooking spray and bake at 450 degrees F for 15 minutes.
3. Position the meatballs on a platter and serve as a snack.

Yogurt Dip

Preparation Time: 10 Minutes
Cooking Time: 0 Minutes
Servings: 6
Nutrition:
Calories: 294,
Fat: 18,
Fiber: 1,
Carbs: 21,
Protein: 10
Ingredients:

- 2 cups Greek yogurt
- 2 tablespoons pistachios, toasted and chopped
- A pinch of salt and white pepper
- 2 tablespoons mint, chopped
- 1 tablespoon kalamata olives, pitted and chopped
- ¼ cup za'atar spice

- ¼ cup pomegranate seeds
- 1/3 cup olive oil

Directions:

1. In a bowl, blend the yogurt with the pistachios and the rest of the ingredients, whisk well.
2. Divide into small cups and serve with pita chips on the side.

Red Pepper Tapenade

Preparation Time: 10 Minutes
Cooking Time: 0 Minutes
Servings: 4
Nutrition:
Calories: 200,
Fat: 5.6,
Fiber: 4.5,
Carbs: 12.4,
Protein: 4.6
Ingredients:

- 7 ounces roasted red peppers, chopped
- ½ cup parmesan, grated
- 1/3 cup parsley, chopped
- 14 ounces canned artichokes, drained and chopped
- 3 tablespoons olive oil
- ¼ cup capers, drained
- 1 and ½ tablespoons lemon juice
- 2 garlic cloves, minced

Directions:

1. In your blender, combine the red peppers with the parmesan and the rest of the ingredients and pulse well.
2. Divide into cups and serve as a snack.

Tomato Bruschetta

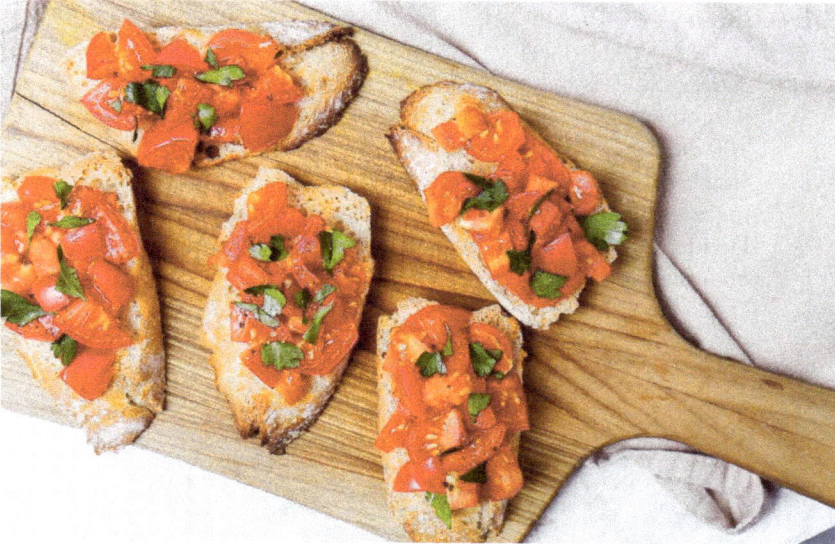

Preparation Time: 10 Minutes
Cooking Time: 10 Minutes
Servings: 6
Nutrition:
Calories: 162,
Fat: 4,
Fiber: 7,
Carbs: 29,
Protein: 4

Ingredients:

- 1 baguette, sliced
- 1/3 cup basil, chopped
- 6 tomatoes, cubed
- 2 garlic cloves, minced
- A pinch of salt and black pepper
- 1 teaspoon olive oil
- 1 tablespoon balsamic vinegar
- ½ teaspoon garlic powder
- Cooking spray

Directions:

1. Arrange the baguette slices in the baking sheet lined with parchment paper, grease them with cooking spray and bake at 400 degrees F for 10 minutes.
2. In a bowl, mix the tomatoes with the basil and the remaining ingredients, toss well and leave aside for 10 minutes.
3. Divide the tomato mix on each baguette slice, arrange them all on a platter and serve.

Artichoke Flatbread

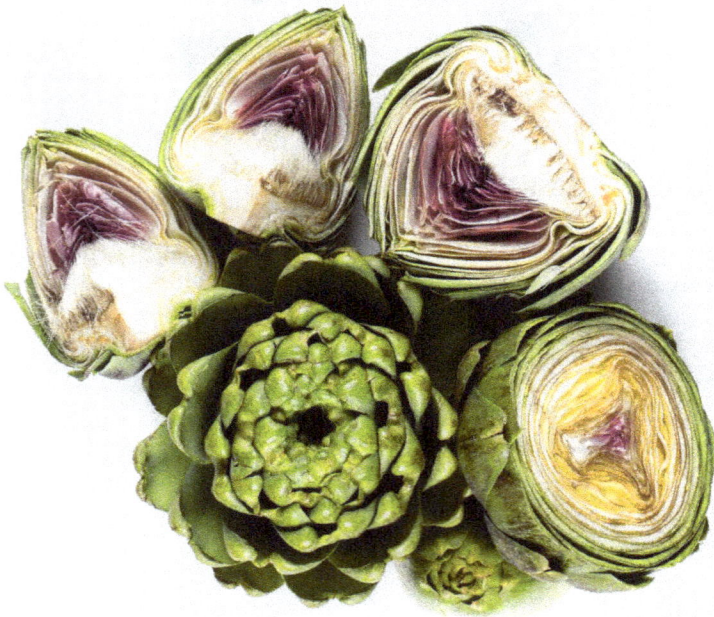

Preparation Time: 10 Minutes
Cooking Time: 15 Minutes
Servings: 4

Nutrition:
Calories: 223,

Fat: 11.2,
Fiber: 5.34,
Carbs: 15.5,
Protein: 7.4

Ingredients:

- 5 tablespoons olive oil
- 2 garlic cloves, minced
- 2 tablespoons parsley, chopped
- 2 round whole wheat flatbreads
- 4 tablespoons parmesan, grated
- $\frac{1}{2}$ cup mozzarella cheese, grated
- 14 ounces canned artichokes, drained and quartered
- 1 cup baby spinach, chopped
- $\frac{1}{2}$ cup cherry tomatoes, halved
- $\frac{1}{2}$ teaspoon basil, dried
- Salt and black pepper to the taste

Directions:

1. In a bowl, mix the parsley with the garlic and 4 tablespoons oil, whisk well and spread this over the flatbreads.
2. Sprinkle the mozzarella and half of the parmesan.
3. In a bowl, mix the artichokes with the spinach, tomatoes, basil, salt, pepper and the rest of the oil, toss and divide over the flatbreads as well.
4. Sprinkle the remaining of the parmesan on top, arrange the flatbreads on a baking sheet lined with parchment paper and bake at 425 degrees F for 15 minutes.
5. Serve a snack.

Coriander Falafel

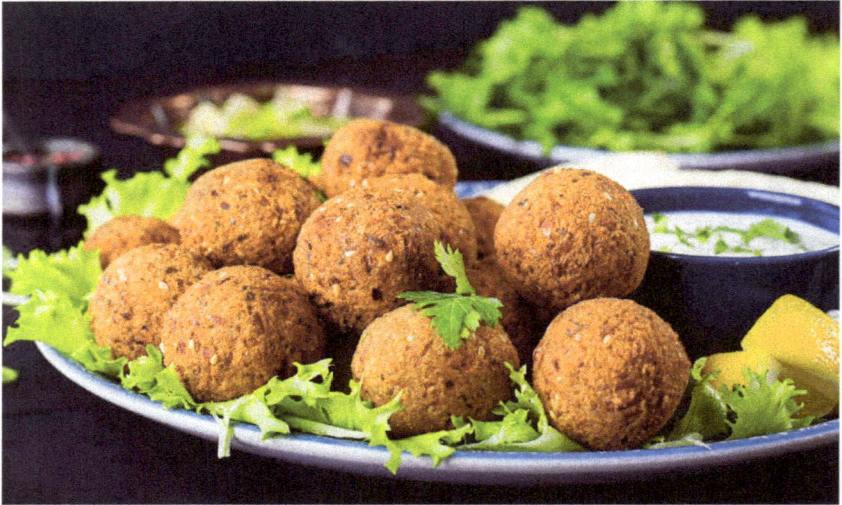

Preparation Time: 10 Minutes
Cooking Time: 10 Minutes
Servings: 8

Nutrition:
Calories: 112,
Fat: 6.2,
Fiber: 2,
Carbs: 12.3
Protein: 3.1
Ingredients:

- 1 cup canned garbanzo beans, drained and rinsed
- 1 bunch parsley leaves
- 1 yellow onion, chopped
- 5 garlic cloves, minced
- 1 teaspoon coriander, ground
- A pinch of salt and black pepper
- ¼ teaspoon cayenne pepper
- ¼ teaspoon baking soda
- ¼ teaspoon cumin powder
- 1 teaspoon lemon juice
- 3 tablespoons tapioca flour

- Olive oil for frying

Directions:

1. In your food processor, combine the beans with the parsley, onion and the rest the ingredients except the oil and the flour and pulse well.
2. Transfer the mix to a bowl, add the flour, stir well, shape 16 balls out of this mix and flatten them a bit.
3. Heat up a pan with some oil over medium-high heat, add the falafels, cook them for 5 minutes on each side, transfer to paper towels, drain excess grease, arrange them on a platter and serve as an appetizer.

Red Pepper Hummus

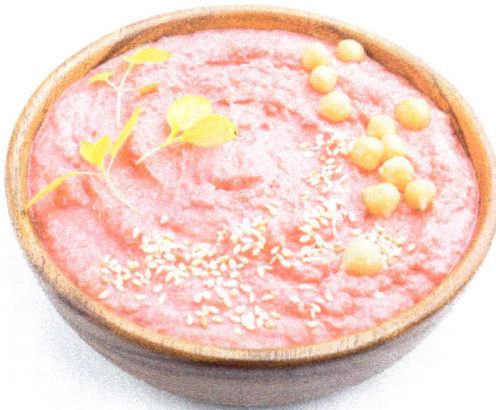

Preparation Time: 10 Minutes
Cooking Time: 0 Minutes
Servings: 6
Nutrition:
Calories: 255,
Fat: 11.4,
Fiber: 4.5,
Carbs: 17.4,

Protein: 6.5

Ingredients:

- 6 ounces roasted red peppers, peeled and chopped
- 16 ounces canned chickpeas, drained and rinsed
- ¼ cup Greek yogurt
- 3 tablespoons tahini paste
- Juice of 1 lemon
- 3 garlic cloves, minced
- 1 tablespoon olive oil
- A pinch of salt and black pepper
- 1 tablespoon parsley, chopped

Directions:

1. In your food processor, combine the red peppers with the rest of the ingredients except the oil and the parsley and pulse well.
2. Add the oil, pulse again, divide into cups, sprinkle the parsley on top and serve as a party spread.

White Bean Dip

Preparation Time: 10 Minutes
Cooking Time: 0 Minutes
Servings: 4
Nutrition:
Calories: 274,
Fat: 11.7,
Fiber: 6.5,
Carbs: 18.5,
Protein: 16.5
Ingredients:

- 15 ounces canned white beans
- 6 ounces canned artichoke hearts, drained and quartered
- 4 garlic cloves, minced
- 1 tablespoon basil, chopped
- 2 tablespoons olive oil

- Juice of ½ lemon
- Zest of ½ lemon, grated
- Salt and black pepper to the taste

Directions:

1. In your food processor, combine the beans with the artichokes and the rest of the ingredients except the oil and pulse well.
2. Add the oil gradually, pulse the mix again, divide into cups and serve as a party dip.

Hummus with Ground Lamb

Preparation Time: 10 Minutes
Cooking Time: 15 Minutes
Servings: 8
Nutrition:
Calories: 133,
Fat: 9.7,
Fiber: 1.7,
Carbs: 6.4,
Protein: 5.4
Ingredients:

- 10 ounces hummus
- 12 ounces lamb meat, ground
- ½ cup pomegranate seeds
- ¼ cup parsley, chopped
- 1 tablespoon olive oil
- Pita chips for serving

Directions:

1. Heat up a pan with the oil over medium-high heat, add the meat, and brown for 15 minutes stirring often.
2. Spread the hummus on a platter, spread the ground lamb all over, also spread the pomegranate seeds and the parsley and serve with pita chips as a snack.

Bulgur Lamb Meatballs

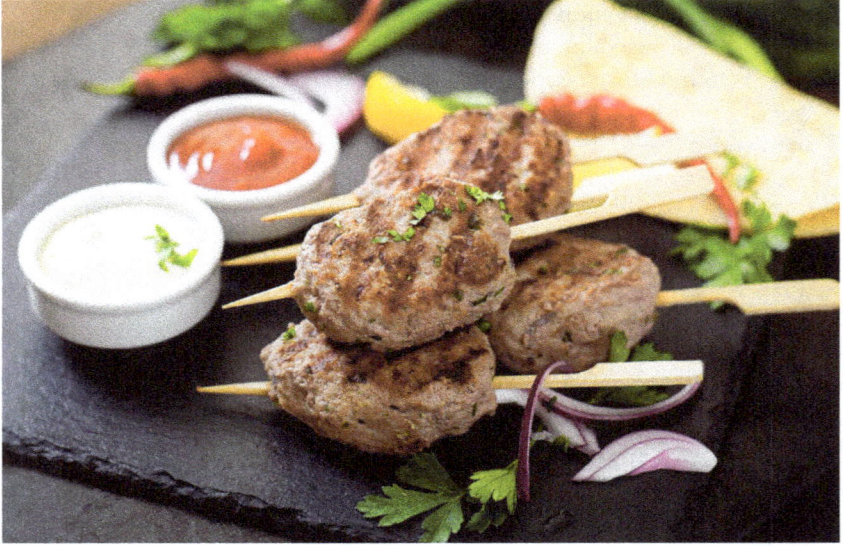

Preparation Time: 10 Minutes
Cooking Time: 15 Minutes
Servings: 6
Nutrition:
Calories: 300,
Fat: 9.6,
Fiber: 4.6,
Carbs: 22.6,
Protein: 6.6

Ingredients:

- 1 and ½ cups Greek yogurt
- ½ teaspoon cumin, ground
- 1 cup cucumber, shredded
- ½ teaspoon garlic, minced
- A pinch of salt and black pepper
- 1 cup bulgur
- 2 cups water
- 1-pound lamb, ground
- ¼ cup parsley, chopped
- ¼ cup shallots, chopped

- ½ teaspoon allspice, ground
- ½ teaspoon cinnamon powder
- 1 tablespoon olive oil

Directions:

1. In a bowl, blend the bulgur with the water, cover the bowl, leave aside for 10 minutes, drain and transfer to a bowl.
2. Add the meat, the yogurt and the rest of the ingredients except the oil, stir well and shape medium meatballs out of this mix.
3. Heat up a pan with the oil over medium-high heat, add the meatballs, cook them for 7 minutes on each side, arrange them all on a platter and serve as a snack.

Eggplant Dip

Preparation Time: 10 Minutes
Cooking Time: 40 Minutes
Servings: 4
Nutrition:
Calories: 121,
Fat: 4.3,
Fiber: 1,
Carbs: 1.4,
Protein: 4.3
Ingredients:

- 1 eggplant, poked with a fork
- 2 tablespoons tahini paste
- 2 tablespoons lemon juice
- 2 garlic cloves, minced
- 1 tablespoon olive oil
- Salt and black pepper to the taste
- 1 tablespoon parsley, chopped

Directions:

1. Put the eggplant in a roasting pan, bake at 400 degrees F for 40 minutes, cool down, peel and transfer to your food processor.
2. Add the rest of the fixings excluding the parsley, pulse well,

divide into small bowls and serve as a snack with the parsley sprinkled on top.

Cucumber Bites

Preparation Time: 10 Minutes
Cooking Time: 0 Minutes
Servings: 12
Nutrition:
Calories: 162,
Fat: 3.4,
Fiber: 2,
Carbs: 6.4,
Protein: 2.4
Ingredients:

- 1 English cucumber, sliced into 32 rounds
- 10 ounces hummus
- 16 cherry tomatoes, halved
- 1 tablespoon parsley, chopped
- 1-ounce feta cheese, crumbled

Directions:

1. Spread the hummus on each cucumber round, divide the tomato halves on each, sprinkle the cheese and parsley on to and serve as a snack.

Veggie Fritters

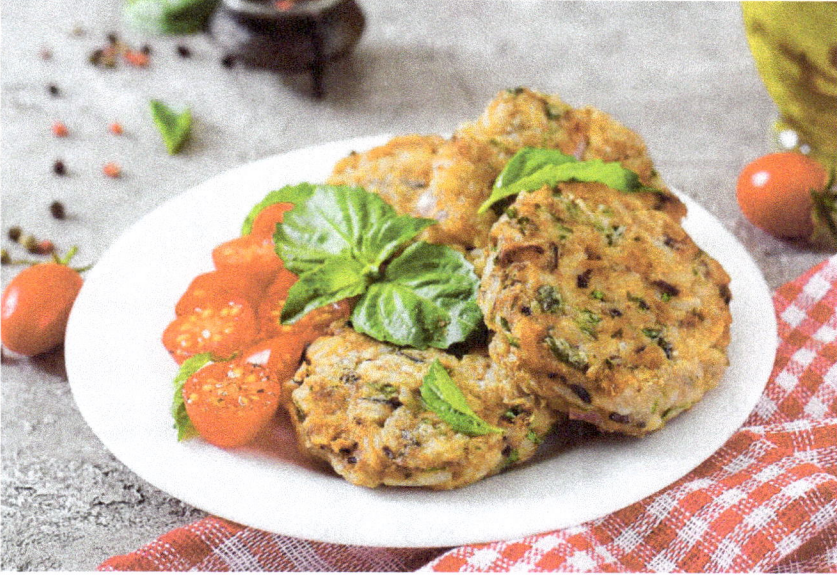

Preparation Time: 10 Minutes
Cooking Time: 10 Minutes
Servings: 8
Nutrition:
Calories: 209,
Fat: 11.2,
Fiber: 3,
Carbs: 4.4,
Protein: 4.8

Ingredients:

- 2 garlic cloves, minced
- 2 yellow onions, chopped
- 4 scallions, chopped
- 2 carrots, grated
- 2 teaspoons cumin, ground
- ½ teaspoon turmeric powder
- Salt and black pepper to the taste
- ¼ teaspoon coriander, ground
- 2 tablespoons parsley, chopped

- ¼ teaspoon lemon juice
- ½ cup almond flour
- 2 beets, peeled and grated
- 2 eggs, whisked
- ¼ cup tapioca flour
- 3 tablespoons olive oil

Directions:

1. In a bowl, combine the garlic with the onions, scallions and the rest of the ingredients except the oil, stir well and shape medium fritters out of this mix.
2. Heat up a pan with the oil on medium-high heat, add the fritters, cook for 5 minutes on each side, arrange on a platter and serve.

Stuffed Avocado

Preparation Time: 10 Minutes
Cooking Time: 0 Minutes
Servings: 2
Nutrition:
Calories: 233,
Fat: 9,
Fiber: 3.5,
Carbs: 11.4,
Protein: 5.6
Ingredients:

- 1 avocado, halved and pitted
- 10 ounces canned tuna, drained
- 2 tablespoons sun-dried tomatoes, chopped
- 1 and ½ tablespoon basil pesto
- 2 tablespoons black olives, pitted and chopped
- Salt and black pepper to the taste
- 2 teaspoons pine nuts, toasted and chopped
- 1 tablespoon basil, chopped

Directions:

1. In a bowl, blend the tuna with the sun-dried tomatoes and the rest of the ingredients except the avocado and stir.
2. Stuff the avocado halves with the tuna mix and serve as a snack.

Wrapped Plums

Preparation Time: 5 Minutes
Cooking Time: 0 Minutes
Servings: 8
Nutrition:
Calories: 30,
Fat: 1,
Fiber: 0,
Carbs: 4,
Protein: 2
Ingredients:

- 2 ounces prosciutto, cut into 16 pieces
- 4 plums, quartered
- 1 tablespoon chives, chopped
- A pinch of red pepper flakes, crushed

Directions:

1. Wrap each plum quarter in a prosciutto slice, arrange them all on a platter, sprinkle the chives and pepper flakes all over and serve.

Cucumber Sandwich Bites

Preparation Time: 5 Minutes
Cooking Time: 0 Minutes
Servings: 12
Nutrition:
Calories: 187
Fat: 12.4
Fiber: 2.1
Carbs: 4.5
Protein: 8.2
Ingredients:

- 1 cucumber, sliced
- 8 slices whole wheat bread
- 2 tablespoons cream cheese, soft
- 1 tablespoon chives, chopped
- ¼ cup avocado, peeled, pitted and mashed
- 1 teaspoon mustard
- Salt and black pepper to the taste

Directions:

1. Spread the mashed avocado on each bread slice, also spread the rest of the ingredients except the cucumber slices.
2. Divide the cucumber slices on the bread slices, cut each slice in thirds, arrange on a platter and serve as a snack.

Cucumber Rolls

Preparation Time: 5 Minutes
Cooking Time: 0 Minutes
Servings: 6
Nutrition:
Calories: 200,
Fat: 6,
Fiber: 3.4,
Carbs: 7.6,
Protein: 3.5
Ingredients:

- 1 big cucumber, sliced lengthwise
- 1 tablespoon parsley, chopped
- 8 ounces canned tuna, drained and mashed
- Salt and black pepper to the taste
- 1 teaspoon lime juice

Directions:

1. Arrange cucumber slices on a working surface, divide the rest of the ingredients, and roll.
2. Arrange all the rolls on a platter and serve as a snack.

Olives and Cheese Stuffed Tomatoes

Preparation Time: 10 Minutes
Cooking Time: 0 Minutes
Servings: 24
Nutrition:
Calories: 136,
Fat: 8.6,
Fiber: 4.8,
Carbs: 5.6,
Protein: 5.1
Ingredients:

- 24 cherry tomatoes, top cut off and insides scooped out
- 2 tablespoons olive oil
- ¼ teaspoon red pepper flakes
- ½ cup feta cheese, crumbled
- 2 tablespoons black olive paste
- ¼ cup mint, torn

Directions:

1. In a bowl, mix the olives paste with the rest of the ingredients except the cherry tomatoes and whisk well.
2. Stuff the cherry tomatoes with this mix, arrange them all on a platter and serve as a snack.

Vinegar Beet Bites

Preparation Time: 10 Minutes
Cooking Time: 30 Minutes
Servings: 4
Nutrition:
Calories: 199,
Fat: 5.4,
Fiber: 3.5,
Carbs: 8.5,
Protein: 3.5
Ingredients:

- 2 beets, sliced
- Sea salt and black pepper

- 1/3 cup balsamic vinegar
- 1 cup olive oil

Directions:

1. Spread the beet slices on a baking sheet lined with parchment paper, add the rest of the ingredients, toss and bake at 350 degrees F for 30 minutes.
2. Serve the beet bites cold as a snack.

Lentils Stuffed Potato Skins

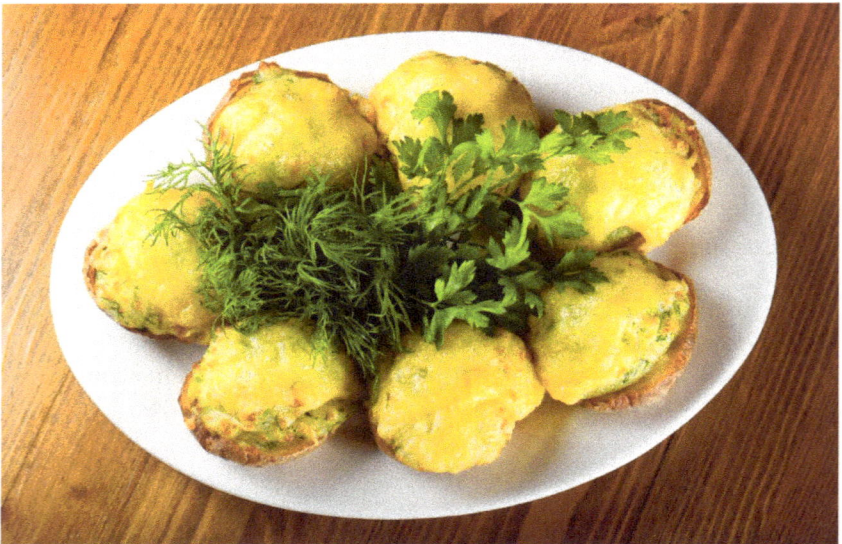

Preparation Time: 10 Minutes
Cooking Time: 30 Minutes
Servings: 8
Nutrition:
Calories: 300,
Fat: 9.3,
Fiber: 14.5,
Carbs: 22.5,
Protein: 8.5

Ingredients:

- 16 red baby potatoes
- ¾ cup red lentils, cooked and drained
- 2 tablespoons olive oil
- 2 garlic cloves, minced
- 1 tablespoon chives, chopped
- ½ teaspoon hot chili sauce
- Salt and black pepper to the taste

Directions:

1. Put potatoes in a pot, add water to cover them, bring to a boil over medium low heat, cook for 15 minutes, drain, cool them down, cut in halves, remove the pulp, transfer it to a blender and pulse it a bit.
2. Add the rest of the ingredients to the blender, pulse again well and stuff the potato skins with this mix.
3. Arrange the stuffed potatoes on a baking sheet lined with parchment paper, introduce them in the oven at 375 degrees F and bake for 15 minutes.
4. Arrange on a platter and serve as an appetizer.

Snacks

Zucchini Pecan Muffins

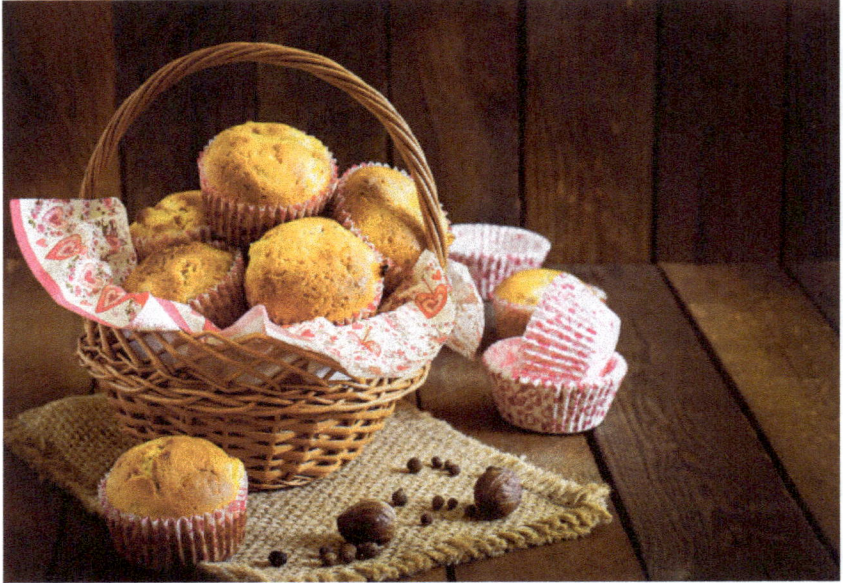

These zucchini pecan muffins give you two out of your five recommended fruit and vegetable servings for the day. They make for a moist, delicious, low-protein snack that can be enjoyed late morning or afternoon to keep your energy going for the day.

Time: 35 minutes

Serving Size: 12

Prep Time: 15 minutes

Cook Time: 20 minutes

Nutritional Info:

Calories: 227

Carbs: 25.6 g

Fat: 13 g

Protein: 2.9 g

Sodium: 212.2 mg

Potassium: 212.2 mg

Phosphorus: 173 mg

Ingredients:

- 1 egg
- 1 ½ cups of flour (all-purpose)
- 1 cup of zucchini (shredded)
- ½ cup of white sugar
- ½ cup of olive oil

- ½ fresh blueberries
- ½ cup of pecans (chopped)
- ¼ cup of brown sugar
- ¼ cup of milk
- 1 ½ tsp of vanilla extract
- 1 tsp of cinnamon
- 1 tsp of baking soda

Directions:

1. Preheat the oven to 350°F, and line 12 muffin cups with paper cups.
2. Combine the dry ingredients in a medium bowl, including the flour, brown sugar, white sugar, baking soda, cinnamon, and salt.
3. Once the dry ingredients are combined, mix together the milk, egg, vanilla extract, and olive oil in a separate bowl until you've reached a smooth consistency.
4. Stir the wet mixture into the dry flour mixture until you've reached a batter consistency.
5. Add the blueberries, shredded zucchini, and pecans to the batter. Fill the muffin cups 2/3 full.
6. Bake the muffins in the preheated oven for 20 to 25 minutes until cooked through. Test this by inserting a toothpick into the muffin, and checking if it comes out clean.

Tortilla Chips and Dip

This snack is nice for when you are looking for something crispy to nibble on before lunch or dinner. It is very low in sodium, protein, fat, potassium, and phosphorus, which means that it ticks all the right boxes to support your kidney condition.

Time: 30 minutes
Serving Size: 4
Prep Time: 20 minutes
Cook Time: 10 minutes
Nutritional Info:
Calories: 56
Carbs: 10 g
Fat: 1 g
Protein: 2 g
Sodium: 81 mg
Potassium: 74 mg
Phosphorus: 48 mg

Ingredients:
- 2 cups of chopped fresh pineapple
- 2 8" whole-wheat tortillas (cut into wedges, rounds, or strips)
- ½ cup of red sweet pepper (finely chopped)
- 1 green onion (sliced)
- 1 tbsp of fresh cilantro (finely chopped)

Directions:

1. Preheat the oven to 375°F.
2. Arrange the tortilla wedges in a single layer onto a large baking sheet, and coat it lightly with cooking spray.
3. Bake the tortilla wedges for 10 minutes until they are golden brown and crisp. Once done, set them aside to cool down, then store them in a sealed container. The wedges should be stored at room temperature and should be consumed within 3 days.
4. Stir together the pineapple, sweet pepper, lime juice, green onion, and cilantro in a medium bowl, and cover it to chill for 24 to 48 hours.
5. Serve the tortilla wedges with a low-sodium dip of your choice, with a side of the fruit and vegetable mix.

Food-prep tip: Seal the tortilla chips in a Ziploc bag for up to 3 days. Enjoy it with a fresh, low-sodium dip in moderation.

Sweet and Savory Popcorn

With only 2 g of protein per serving, this sweet and savory snack is ideal for a variety of kidney conditions. It is gluten-free, and can be served seasoned or unseasoned.

Time: 5 minutes
Serving Size: 2 cups
Prep Time: 0 minutes
Cook Time: 5 minutes
Nutritional Info:
Calories: 120
Carbs: 12 g
Fat: 7 g
Protein: 2 g
Sodium: 2 mg
Potassium: 56 mg
Phosphorus: 60 mg
Ingredients:
- 8 cups of popcorn (air-popped)
- 2 tbsp of butter (unsalted)

- 2 tbsp of brown sugar
- ½ tsp of cinnamon
- ¼ tsp of nutmeg

Directions:

1. Heat the butter, cinnamon, brown sugar, and nutmeg over medium heat in a saucepan until the sugar melts and dissolves. Alternatively, the ingredients can be microwaved but should be monitored so that the butter doesn't burn.
2. Drizzle the spiced butter mixture over the popped popcorn. Mix the ingredients well before serving.

Food-prep tip: Preserve the coated popcorn in Ziploc bags for individual on-the-go servings. Store them a room temperature for up to 5 days.

Pumpkin Spice Yogurt

Whether it's Halloween or not, you get to enjoy spiced yogurt for a snack at any time of the year. Not only is this snack low in calories, but it can give you your calcium fix, boost your immune system, and make you feel like you're having dessert when you're sticking to a healthy, balanced diet. If you're not the meal-prep type, this snack is especially for you as it can be prepared in under five minutes.

Time: 3 minutes
Serving Size: 1
Prep Time: 3 minutes
Cook Time: 0 minutes
Nutritional Info:
Calories: 149
Carbs: 8 g
Fat: 4.2 g
Protein: 20 g
Sodium: 65.6 mg
Potassium: 35.75 mg
Phosphorus: 24.6 mg

Ingredients:

- 7 oz of plain Greek yogurt
- 1 tbsp of pumpkin puree
- ¼ tsp of cinnamon
- ¼ tsp of nutmeg
- ¼ tsp of honey

Directions:

1. Place the ingredients in a bowl and stir them together until they are well combined.
2. Serve the yogurt immediately, or store it in the refrigerator in an airtight container.

Food-prep tip: Make two to five servings more and store them in individual containers to take with you on the go. Keep the yogurt in the refrigerator for up to 5 days for a daily snack when you're tight on time.

Rosemary Roasted Almonds

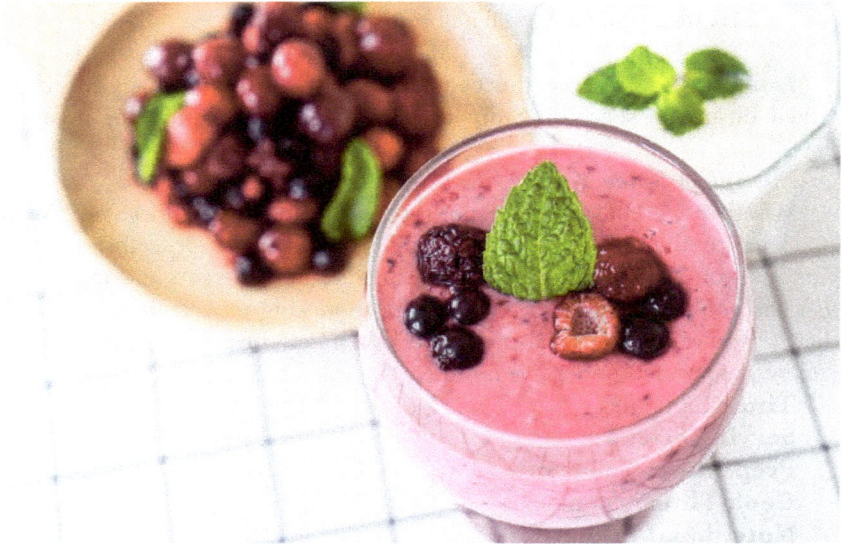

As a source of healthy fats and Omega-3s, and serving as a savory snack, these roasted almonds are ideal for keeping you fuller for longer to prevent overeating and support weight loss. It can be prepped for a snack for the entire week and is quick and easy to make for a good source of protein appropriate for those with reduced kidney function.

Time: 25 minutes
Serving Size: 8
Prep Time: 5 minutes
Cook Time: 20 minutes
Nutritional Info:
Calories: 355
Carbs: 13 g
Fat: 31 g
Protein: 13 g

Sodium:223 mg

Potassium: 451 mg

Phosphorus: 298 mg

Ingredients:

- 2 cups of almonds (whole)
- 1 tbsp of olive oil
- 1 tbsp of rosemary (fresh, finely chopped)
- 1 sp of chili powder
- ¾ tsp of Himalayan salt
- ¼ tsp of cayenne pepper

Directions:

1. Preheat the oven to 325°F.
2. Combine the almonds, olive oil, rosemary, chili powder, Himalayan salt, and cayenne pepper in a small bowl.
3. Stir the ingredients well to coat the almonds.
4. Line a baking sheet with parchment paper and arrange the almonds with space between each. Bake them for 20 minutes before removing them from the oven.

Food-prep tip: Once cooled down, store the almonds in a Ziploc bag or sealed plastic container at room temperature or in the refrigerator for up to 5 days.

Berry Smoothie

For a delicious ice-cold smoothie, blend a variety of berries, including raspberries, blueberries, strawberries, and blackberries, to get an antioxidant and immune boost. This smoothie is low in calories, carbs, fat, and contains a good source of protein. It is also very low in sodium to support kidney function.

Time: 2 minutes

Serving Size: 2 (7 oz per serving)

Prep Time: 2 minutes

Cook Time: 0 minutes

Nutritional Info:

Calories: 152

Carbs: 15 g

Fat: 4 g

Protein: 14 g

Sodium: 84 mg

Potassium: 216 mg

Phosphorus: 76 mg

Ingredients:

- 4 oz of water (cold)
- 1 cup of frozen mixed berries
- ½ cup of coconut cream
- 1 tsp of berry maca powder
- 2 scoops of whey protein

Directions:

1. Add the frozen berries, water, and maca powder to the blender, and blend the ingredients at medium speed until they are mixed well.
2. Add coconut cream to the blender and blend to reach a creamy consistency.
3. Add protein powder to the smoothie and blend well.
4. Divide the smoothie into 2 servings, and serve the smoothies chilled right away.

Food-prep tip: Freeze the smoothie in a sealed container for up to 3 days to serve later.

Pumpkin Bread

Sometimes, all you may be craving is a tasty slice of bread. Although bread is limited on the kidney-friendly renal diet, nobody said anything about restricting pumpkin bread!

Time: 1 hour and 20 minutes
Serving Size: 10 (1 slice ¾" thick)
Prep Time: 10 minutes
Cook Time: 70 minutes
Nutritional Info:
Calories: 187
Carbs: 31 g
Fat: 6 g
Protein: 2 g
Sodium: 45 mg
Potassium: 69 mg
Phosphorus: 75 mg

Ingredients:

- 1 eggs
- 1 ¼ cups of flour (all-purpose)
- 1 cups of brown sugar
- ½ can of pumpkin (15 oz)
- ½ cup of whole cranberries (fresh)
- ¼ cup of vegetable oil
- 1 tsp of pumpkin pie spice

- 1 tsp of baking powder

Directions:

1. Preheat the oven to 350°F.
2. In a large bowl, combine the pumpkin pie spice, flour, and baking powder, and mix the dry ingredients well.
3. Add the eggs, pumpkin puree, brown sugar, and vegetable oil to a small mixing bowl, and beat the ingredients until properly blended.
4. Add the pumpkin mixture to the flour mixture, and stir everything until moistened. Continue to beat the mixture with a spoon until you've reached a good consistency without clumps.
5. Spoon the batter into a 9" x 5" loaf pan and bake the bread in the oven for 60 minutes.
6. Remove the pan from the oven, allowing them to cool for 10 minutes before slicing the bread into 10 ¾ inch-thick slices.

Food-prep tip: Store the pumpkin bread (sliced) in an airtight container in the refrigerator for up to 4 days.

Peanut Butter Bars

A little goes a long way. For a sweet and satisfying snack — 10 of them, to be exact — opt for this low-protein and low-carb treat, which contains a low source of sodium, potassium, and phosphorus to support your kidney health. This snack is vegetarian, gluten-free, and heart-healthy.

Time: 70 minutes
Serving Size: 10 (1 bar each)
Prep Time: 10 minutes
Cook Time: 60 minutes
Nutritional Info:
Calories: 275
Carbs: 26 g
Fat: 9 g
Protein: 8 g
Sodium: 102 mg
Potassium: 173 mg
Phosphorus: 120 mg
Ingredients:
- 2 cups of rolled oats
- ½ cup of whey protein powder
- ½ cup of peanut butter (melted)
- ¼ cup of mini dark chocolate chips

- ⅓ cup of honey
- ½ tsp of cinnamon
- ⅛ tsp of Himalayan salt (fine)

Directions:

1. Line a 5" x 8" baking dish with parchment paper.
2. Add the oats, cinnamon, and Himalayan salt to a medium bowl, and mix well.
3. Combine the protein powder, honey, and peanut butter in a medium bowl.
4. Add the wet mixture to the dry mixture, and mix everything until you have a well-blended sticky mixture.
5. Pat the mixture evenly into the lined baking dish, and sprinkle the top with dark chocolate chips. Pat the top of the dish to ensure there is an even layer on top.
6. Refrigerate the mixture for one hour.
7. Once done, remove the mixture from the refrigerator, and cut it into 5 sections. Half the 5 sections into 10 bars in total.

Food-prep tip: Wrap each bar in parchment paper or plastic wrap. Keep them refrigerated until for an on-the-go snack.

Roasted Garbanzo Beans

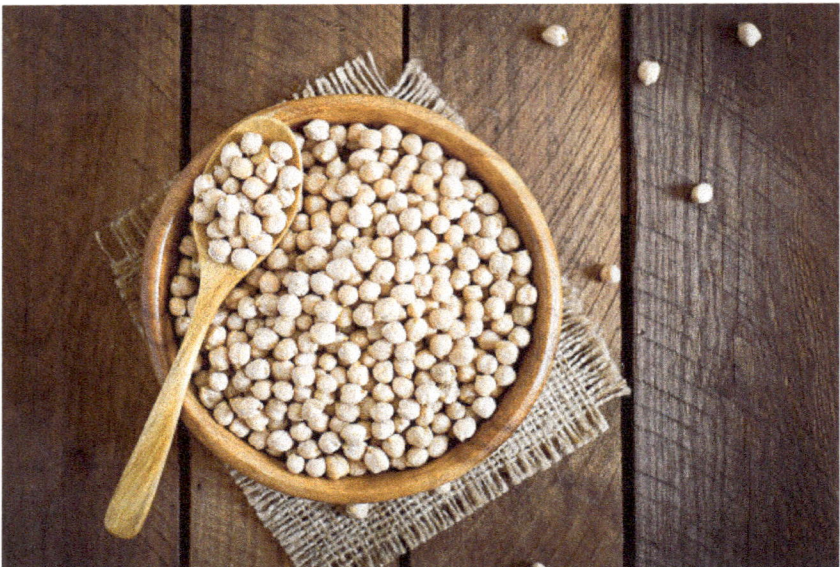

Roasted chickpeas, otherwise known as garbanzo beans, are terrific as a low-protein daily snack, and can also be enjoyed among friends as a light snack before a meal. They can be eaten plain, tossed up with a green salad, added to your favorite trail mix, and packed seasoned in your snack box for a busy day.

Time: 40 minutes
Serving Size: 4
Prep Time: 5 minutes
Cook Time: 35 minutes
Nutritional Info:
Calories: 96
Carbs: 15 g
Fat: 2 g
Protein: 6 g
Sodium: 369 mg
Potassium: 72.5 mg
Phosphorus: 48 mg
Ingredients:
- 15 oz of chickpeas/garbanzo beans (canned)
- 2 tsp of olive oil
- 1 tsp of garlic powder
- ⅛ tsp of kosher salt

Directions:

1. Preheat the oven to 375°F.
2. Drain and rinse the chickpeas, then pat dry them with a paper towel.
3. Arrange the chickpeas on a baking sheet and roast them for 30 minutes, removing the sheet from the oven every ten minutes to give them a good shake. The final product should be crunchy and golden brown, not moist. The chickpeas should be monitored closely to ensure they don't burn.
4. Combine salt and garlic powder in a medium bowl.
5. Remove the chickpeas from the oven once done, and add the olive oil over them immediately. Follow this by tossing the seasoning over them, and shaking them once more.
6. Allow them to cool before serving.

Food-prep tip: Store the chickpeas at room temperature in a Ziploc bag for up to 3 days. Prepare more in advance for snacks for busy weekdays.

Savory Roll Bites
These tasty bites offer a good source of protein and are a great alterna-

tive to the traditional sweet-treat protein balls. With a variety of flavors, it's an exciting snack you can look forward to every day.

Time: 10 minutes

Serving Size: 5 (2 balls per serving)

Prep Time: 10 minutes

Cook Time: 0 minutes

Nutritional Info:

Calories: 310

Carbs: 18.2 g

Fat: 16.8 g

Protein: 14 g

Sodium: 388 mg

Potassium: 205 mg

Phosphorus: 143 mg

Ingredients:

Pizza balls:

- ½ cup of white beans (drained and rinsed)
- ½ cup of almonds
- 2 tbsp of oat flour
- 1 tbsp of tomato paste
- 1 tbsp of nutritional yeast
- ½ tsp of Italian seasoning
- ⅛ tsp of kosher salt

Curry balls:

- ½ cup of white beans (drained and rinsed)
- ½ cup of cashews
- 2 tbsp of oat flour
- ½ tsp of garlic powder
- ½ tsp of curry powder
- ⅛ tsp of kosher salt

Garlic & herb balls:

- ½ cup of white beans (drained and rinsed)
- ¼ cup of tahini
- ¼ cup of oat flour
- ½ tsp of garlic powder
- ½ tsp of Italian seasoning
- ⅛ tsp of kosher salt

Directions:

1. Assemble three different types of balls by combining each set of ingredients separately in the food processor at a high speed. Pulse the ingredients until everything is well-combined. Do this

starting with the pizza balls, followed by the curry balls, and then the garlic & herb balls. Clean the food processor each time after you've blended one type and removed the contents.

2. Wet your fingers a little to prevent the dough from sticking. Use a ½ tbsp measure and scoop out some dough, and then roll it into spheres to create between 10 to 12 balls.

3. Store the savory bites in an airtight container and place them in the refrigerator for up to a week. They can also be frozen for up to 6 weeks.

Food-prep tip: Store the savory bites in individual containers or Ziploc bags to take them on the go during a busy week.

3

Salads

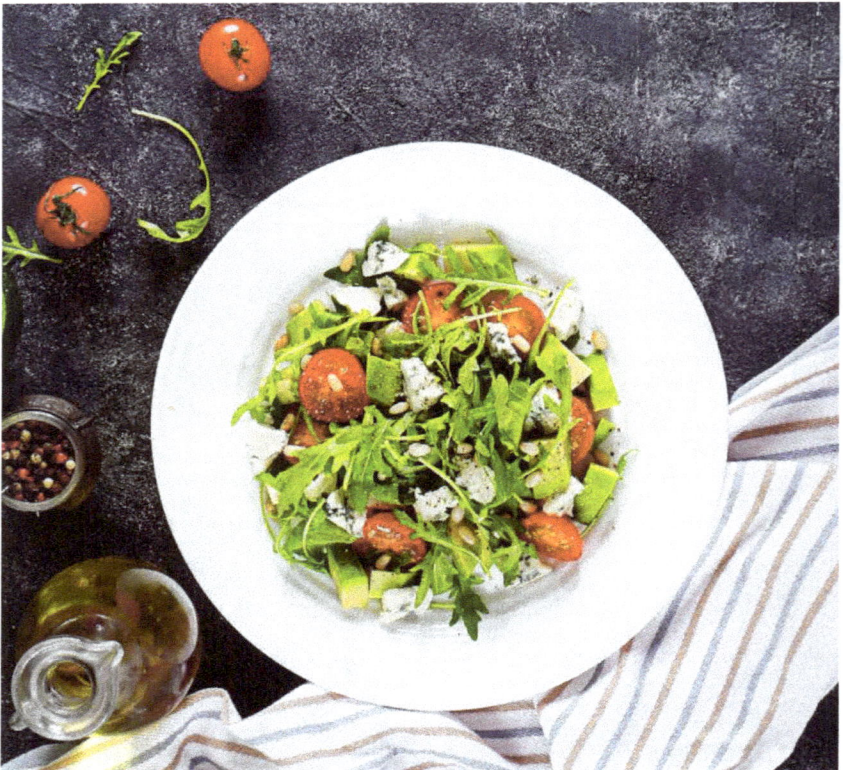

Spelled Salad

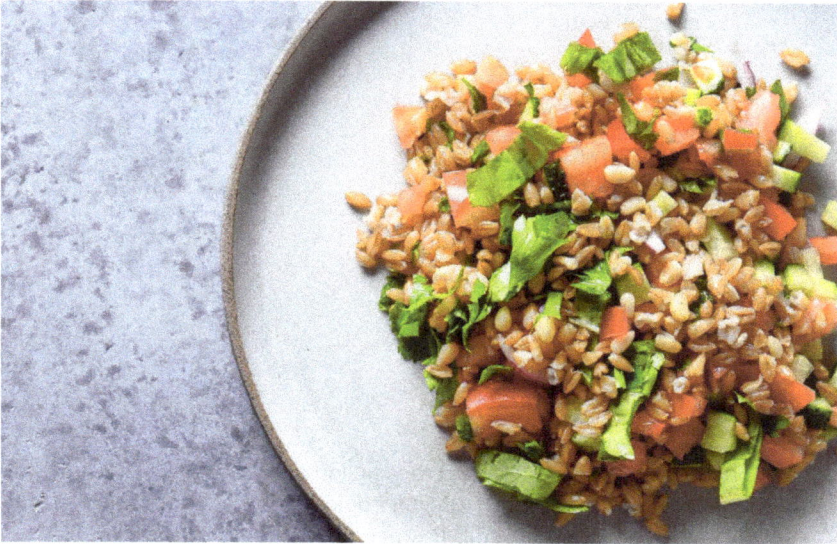

Preparation Time: 15 Minutes
  Cooking Time: 30 Minutes
  Servings: 4
  Nutrition:
  Calories:365
  Fat:10g
  Carbohydrates:43g
  Protein:13g
  Sodium:845mg

Ingredients:

- Salad
- 2 ½ cups of vegetable broth
- ¾ cup of crumbled feta cheese
- 1 can chickpeas, drained
- 1 cucumber, chopped
- 1 ½ cup pearl spelled
- 1 tablespoon of olive oil
- ½ sliced onion

- 2 cups of baby spinach, chopped
- 1 pint of cherry tomatoes
- 1 ¼ cups of water

1. **Dressing:**

- 2 tablespoons of lemon juice
- 1 tablespoon of honey
- ¼ cup olive oil
- ¼ tsp oregano
- 1 pinch of red pepper flakes
- ¼ teaspoon of salt
- 1 tablespoon of red wine vinegar

Directions:

1. Heat the oil in a skillet. Add the spelled and cook for a minute. Be sure to stir it regularly during cooking. Fill in water and broth, then bring to a boil. Reduce the heat and simmer until the spelled is tender, about 30 minutes. Drain the water and transfer the spelled to a bowl.
2. Add the spinach and mix. Let cool for about 20 minutes. Add the cucumber, onions, tomatoes, peppers, chickpeas and feta. Mix well to get a good mixture. Step back and prepare the dressing.
3. Mix all the dressing ingredients and mix well until smooth. Pour it into the bowl and mix it well. Season well to taste.

Chickpea and Zucchini Salad

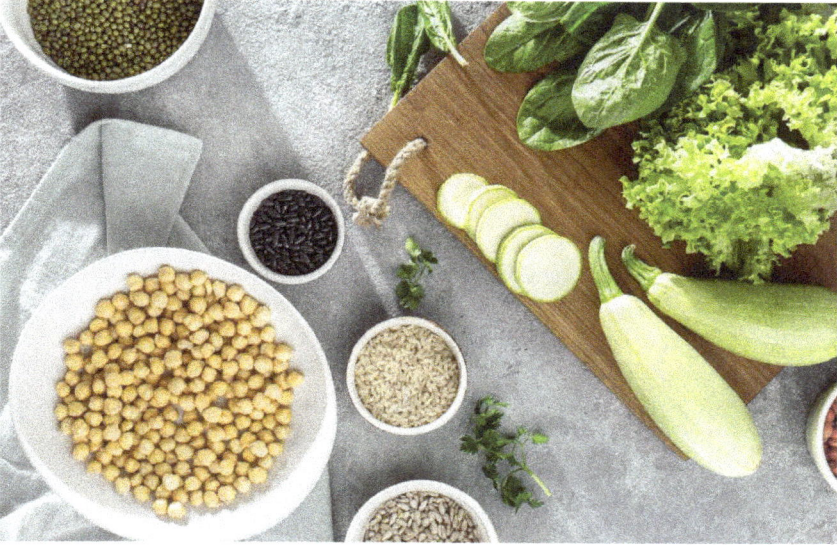

Preparation Time: 10 Minutes
Cooking Time: 0 Minutes
Servings: 3
Nutrition:
Calories:258
Fat:12g
Carbohydrates:19g
Protein:5.6g
Sodium:686mg

Ingredients:

- ¼ cup balsamic vinegar
- 1/3 cup chopped basil leaves
- 1 tablespoon of capers, drained and chopped
- ½ cup crumbled feta cheese
- 1 can chickpeas, drained
- 1 garlic clove, chopped
- ½ cup Kalamata olives, chopped
- 1/3 cup of olive oil
- ½ cup sweet onion, chopped
- ½ tsp oregano

- 1 pinch of red pepper flakes, crushed
- ¾ cup red bell pepper, chopped
- 1 tablespoon chopped rosemary
- 2 cups of zucchini, diced
- salt and pepper, to taste

Directions:

1. Combine the vegetables in a bowl and cover well.
2. Serve at room temperature. But for best results, refrigerate the bowl for a few hours before serving, to allow the flavors to blend.

Provencal Artichoke Salad

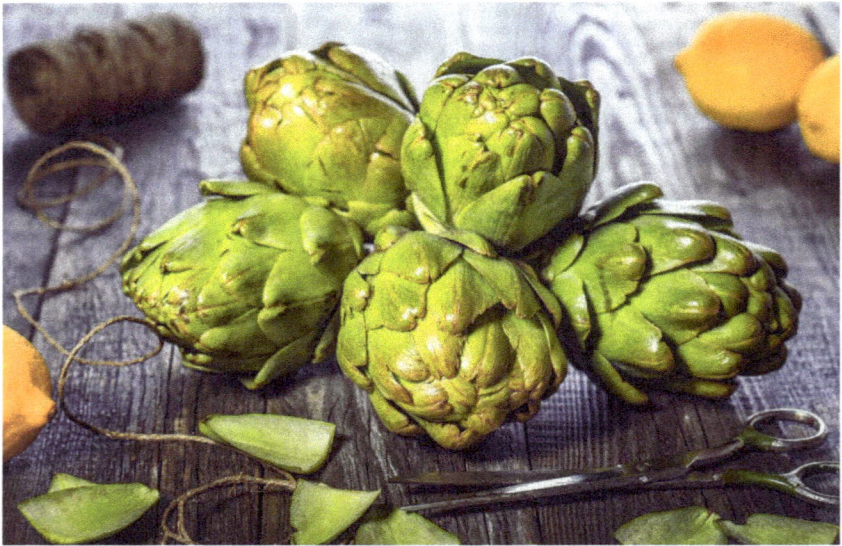

Preparation Time: 15 Minutes
Cooking Time: 5 Minutes
Servings: 3
Nutrition:
Calories:147
Fat:13g
Carbohydrates:18g
Protein:4g
Sodium:689mg

. . .

Ingredients:

- 9 oz artichoke hearts
- 1 teaspoon of chopped basil
- 2 garlic cloves, chopped
- 1 lemon zest
- 1 tablespoon olives, chopped
- 1 tablespoon of olive oil
- ½ chopped onion
- 1 pinch, ½ teaspoon of salt
- 2 tomatoes, chopped
- 3 tablespoons of water
- ½ glass of white wine
- salt and pepper, to taste

Directions:

1. Heat the oil in a skillet. Sauté the onion and garlic. Cook until the onions are translucent and season with a pinch of salt. Pour in the white wine and simmer until the wine is reduced by half.
2. Add the chopped tomatoes, artichoke hearts and water. Simmer then add the lemon zest and about ½ teaspoon of salt. Cover and cook for about 6 minutes.
3. Add the olives and basil. Season well and enjoy!

Bulgarian Salad

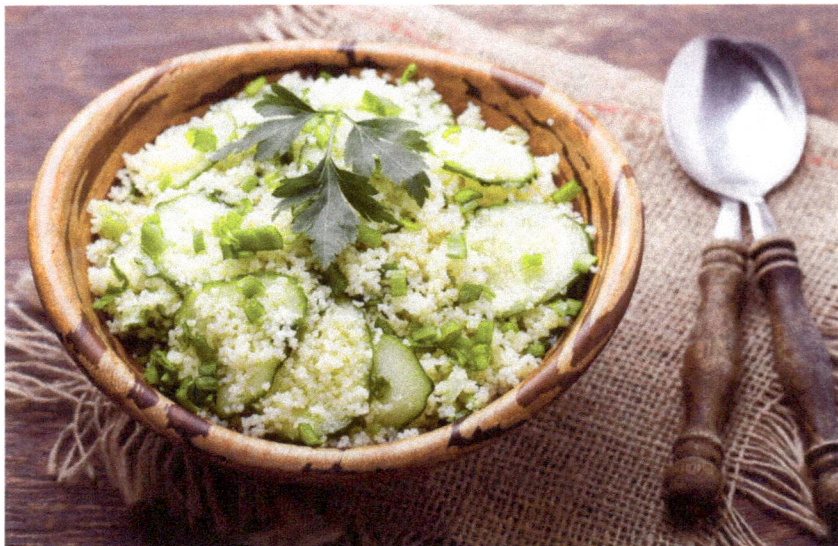

Preparation Time: 10 Minutes
Cooking Time: 20 Minutes
Servings: 2
Nutrition:
Calories:386
Fat:14g
Carbohydrates:55g
Protein:9g
Sodium:545mg

Ingredients:

- 2 cups of bulgur
- 1 tablespoon of butter
- 1 cucumber, cut into pieces
- ¼ cup dill
- ¼ cup black olives, cut in half
- 1 tablespoon, 2 teaspoons of olive oil
- 4 cups of water
- 2 teaspoons of red wine vinegar
- salt, to taste

Directions:

1. In a saucepan, toast the bulgur on a mixture of butter and olive oil. Leave to cook until the bulgur is golden brown and begins to crack.
2. Add water and season with salt. Wrap everything and simmer for about 20 minutes or until the bulgur is tender.
3. In a bowl, mix the cucumber pieces with the olive oil, dill, red wine vinegar and black olives. Mix everything well.
4. It combines cucumber and bulgur.

Falafel Salad Bowl

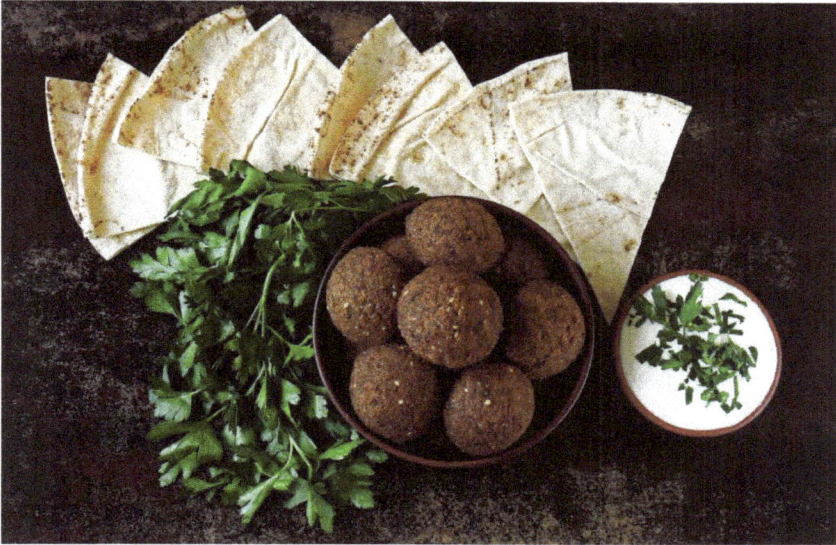

Preparation Time: 15 Minutes
Cooking Time: 5 Minutes
Servings: 2
Nutrition:
Calories:561
Fat:11g
Carbohydrates:60.1g
Protein:18.5g
Sodium:944mg

. . .

Ingredients:

- 1 tablespoon of chili garlic sauce
- 1 tablespoon of garlic and dill sauce
- 1 pack of vegetarian falafels
- 1 box of humus
- 2 tablespoons of lemon juice
- 1 tablespoon of pitted kalamata olives
- 1 tablespoon of extra virgin olive oil
- ¼ cup onion, diced
- 2 cups of chopped parsley
- 2 cups of crisp pita
- 1 pinch of salt
- 1 tablespoon of tahini sauce
- ½ cup diced tomato

Directions:

1. Cook the prepared falafels. Put it aside.
2. Prepare the salad. Mix the parsley, onion, tomato, lemon juice, olive oil and salt. Throw it all out and put everything aside.
3. Transfer everything to the serving bowls.
4. Add the parsley and cover with humus and falafel.
5. Sprinkle bowl with tahini sauce, chili garlic sauce and dill sauce.
6. Upon serving, add the lemon juice and mix the salad well. Serve with pita bread on the side.

Easy Greek Salad

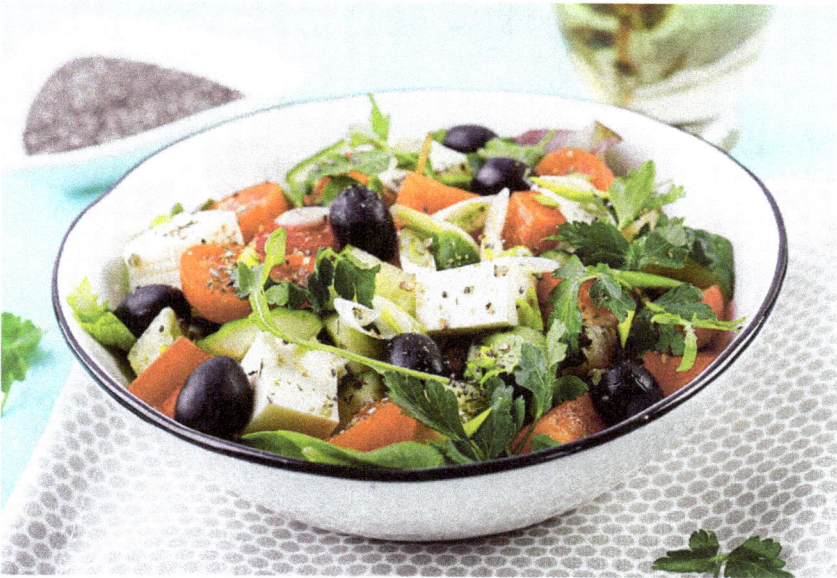

Preparation Time: 15 Minutes
Cooking Time: 0 Minutes
Servings: 2
Nutrition:
Calories:292
Fat:17g
Carbohydrates:12g
Protein:6g
Sodium:743mg

Ingredients:

- 4 oz Greek feta cheese, cubed
- 5 cucumbers, cut lengthwise
- 1 teaspoon of honey
- 1 lemon, chewed and grated
- 1 cup kalamata olives, pitted and halved
- ¼ cup extra virgin olive oil
- 1 onion, sliced
- 1 teaspoon of oregano
- 1 pinch of fresh oregano (for garnish)

- 12 tomatoes, quartered
- ¼ cup red wine vinegar
- salt and pepper, to taste

Directions:

1. In a bowl, soak the onions in salted water for 15 minutes.
2. In a large bowl, combine the honey, lemon juice, lemon peel, oregano, salt and pepper.
3. Mix everything. Gradually add the olive oil, beating as you do, until the oil emulsifies. Add the olives and tomatoes. Put it right. Add the cucumbers
4. Drain the onions soaked in salted water and add them to the salad mixture. Top the salad with fresh oregano and feta. Dash with olive oil and season with pepper, to taste.

Arugula Salad with Figs and Walnuts

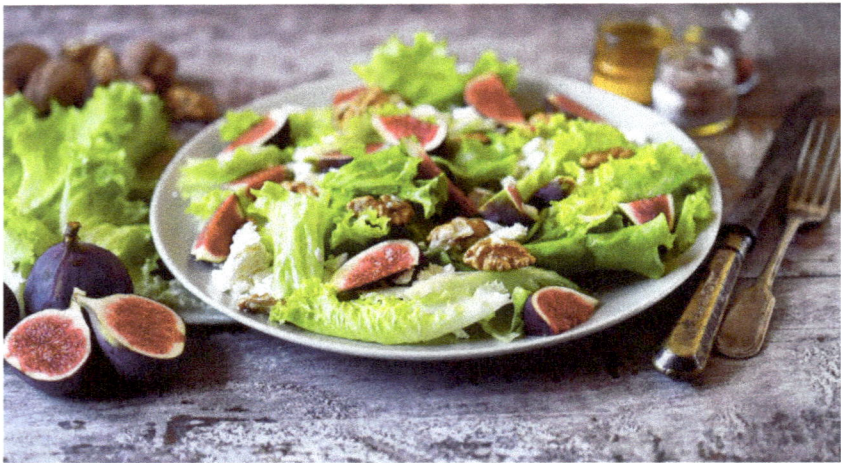

Preparation Time: 15 Minutes
Cooking Time: 10 Minutes
Servings: 2

Nutrition:

Calories:403
Fat:9g

Carbohydrates:35g
Protein:13g
Sodium:844mg

Ingredients:

- 5 oz arugula
- 1 carrot, scraped
- 1/8 teaspoon of cayenne pepper
- 3 oz of goat cheese, crumbled
- 1 can salt-free chickpeas, drained
- ½ cup dried figs, cut into wedges
- 1 teaspoon of honey
- 3 tablespoons of olive oil
- 2 teaspoons of balsamic vinegar
- ½ walnuts cut in half
- salt, to taste

Directions:

1. Preheat the oven to 175 degrees. In a baking dish, combine the nuts, 1 tablespoon of olive oil, cayenne pepper and 1/8 teaspoon of salt. Transfer the baking sheet in the oven and bake it until the nuts are golden. Set it aside when you are done.
2. In a bowl, incorporate the honey, balsamic vinegar, 2 tablespoons of oil and ¾ teaspoon of salt.
3. In a large bowl, combine the arugula, carrot and figs. Add nuts and goat cheese and drizzle with balsamic honey vinaigrette. Make sure you cover everything.

Cauliflower Salad with Tahini Vinaigrette

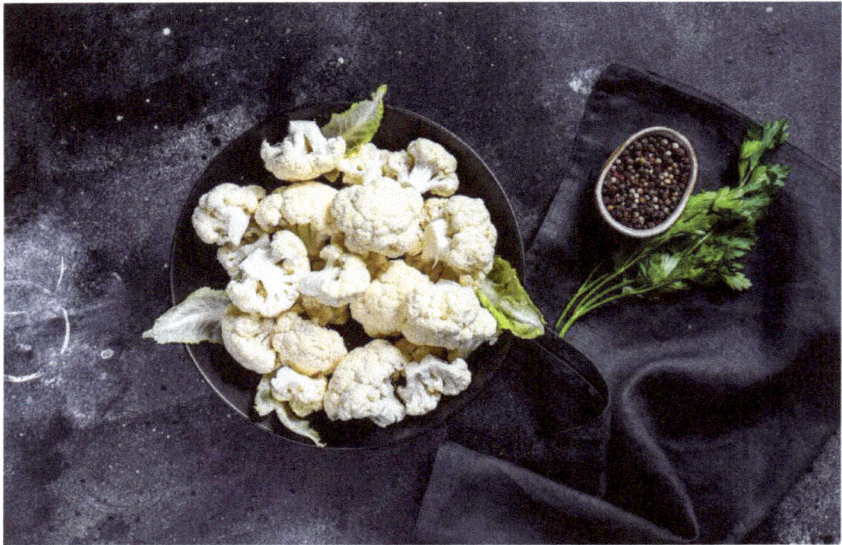

Preparation Time: 15 Minutes
Cooking Time: 5 Minutes
Servings: 2
Nutrition:
Calories:165
Fat:10g
Carbohydrates:20g
Protein:6g
Sodium:651mg
Ingredients:

- 1 ½ lb. of cauliflower
- ¼ cup of dried cherries
- 3 tablespoons of lemon juice
- 1 tablespoon of fresh mint, chopped
- 1 teaspoon of olive oil
- ½ cup chopped parsley
- 3 tablespoons of roasted salted pistachios, chopped
- ½ teaspoon of salt
- ¼ Cup of shallot, chopped
- 2 tablespoons of tahini

Directions:

1. Grate the cauliflower in a microwave-safe container Add olive oil and ¼ salt. Be sure to cover and season the cauliflower evenly. Wrap the bowl with plastic wrap and heat it in the microwave for about 3 minutes.
2. Put the rice with the cauliflower on a baking sheet and let cool for about 10 minutes. Add the lemon juice and the shallots. Let it rest to allow the cauliflower to absorb the flavor.
3. Add the mixture of tahini, cherries, parsley, mint and salt. Mix everything well. Sprinkle with roasted pistachios before serving.

Mediterranean Potato Salad

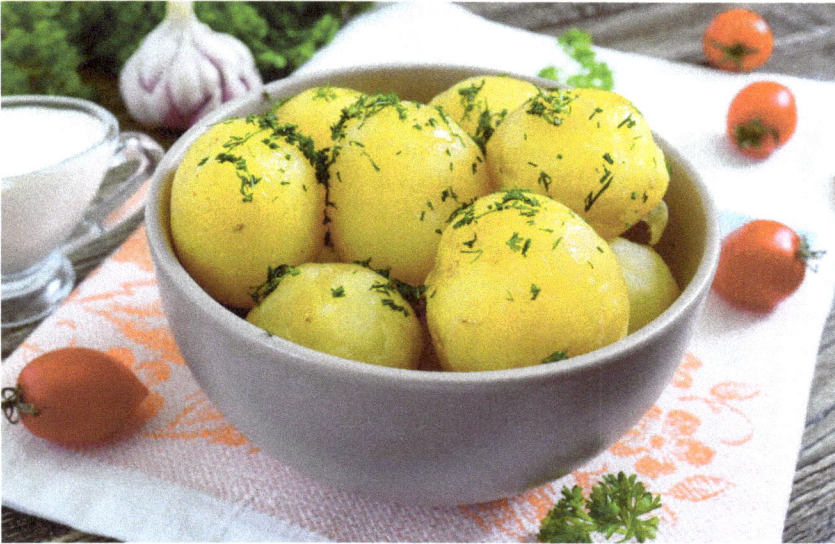

Preparation Time: 15 Minutes
Cooking Time: 10 Minutes
Servings: 2
Nutrition:
Calories:111
Fat:9g
Carbohydrates:16g
Protein:3g
Sodium:745mg

Ingredients:

- 1 bunch of basil leaves, torn
- 1 garlic clove, crushed
- 1 tablespoon of olive oil
- 1 onion, sliced
- 1 teaspoon of oregano
- 100 g of roasted red pepper. Slices
- 300g potatoes, cut in half
- 1 can of cherry tomatoes
- salt and pepper, to taste

Directions:

1. Sauté the onions in a saucepan. Add oregano and garlic. He cooks everything for a minute. Add the pepper and tomatoes. Season well, then simmer for about 10 minutes. Put that aside.
2. In a saucepan, boil the potatoes in salted water. Cook until tender, about 15 minutes. Drain well. Mix the potatoes with the sauce and add the basil and olives. Finally, throw everything away before serving.

Quinoa and Pistachio Salad

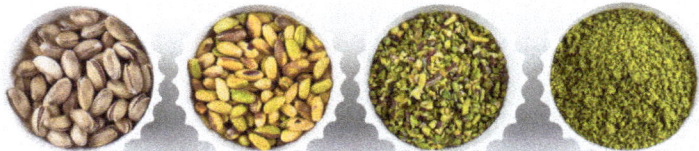

Preparation Time: 10 Minutes
Cooking Time: 15 Minutes
Servings: 2
Nutrition:
Calories:248
Fat:8g
Carbohydrates:35g
Protein:7g
Sodium:914mg

Ingredients:

- ¼ teaspoon of cumin
- ½ cup of dried currants
- 1 teaspoon grated lemon zest
- 2 tablespoons of lemon juice
- ½ cup green onions, chopped
- 1 tablespoon of chopped mint
- 2 tablespoons of extra virgin olive oil
- ¼ cup chopped parsley
- ¼ teaspoon ground pepper
- 1/3 cup pistachios, chopped
- 1 ¼ cups uncooked quinoa
- 1 2/3 cup of water

Directions:

1. In a saucepan, combine 1 2/3 cups of water, raisins and quinoa.
2. Cook everything until boiling then reduce the heat. Simmer everything for about 10 minutes and let the quinoa become frothy. Set it aside for about 5 minutes.
3. In a container, transfer the quinoa mixture. Add the nuts, mint, onions and parsley. Mix everything.
4. In separate bowl, incorporate the lemon zest, lemon juice, currants, cumin and oil. Beat them together. Mix the dry and wet ingredients.

Cucumber Chicken Salad with Spicy Peanut Dressing

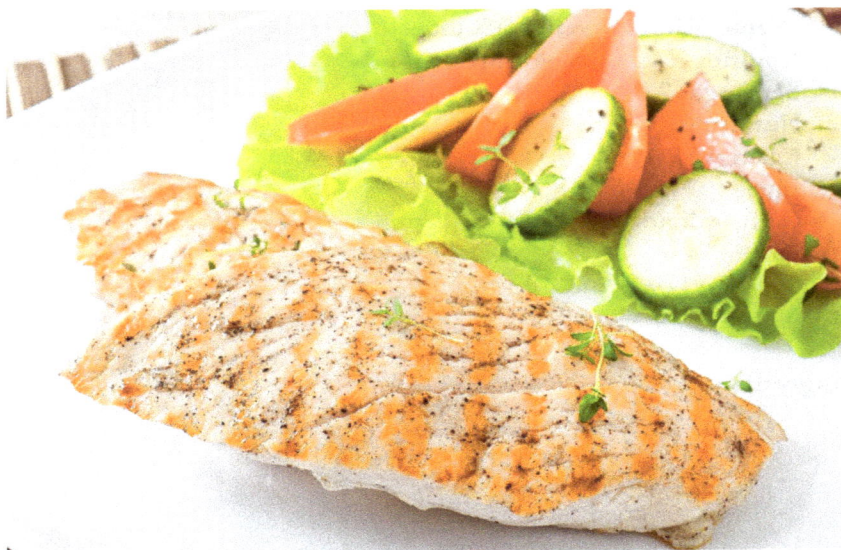

Preparation Time: 15 Minutes
Cooking Time: 0 Minutes
Servings: 2
Nutrition:
720 calories
54 g fat
8.9g carbohydrates
45.9g protein
733mg sodium
Ingredients:

- 1/2 cup peanut butter
- 1 tablespoon sambal oelek (chili paste)
- 1 tablespoon low-sodium soy sauce
- 1 teaspoon grilled sesame oil
- 4 tablespoons of water, or more if necessary
- 1 cucumber with peeled and cut into thin strips
- 1 cooked chicken fillet, grated into thin strips
- 2 tablespoons chopped peanuts

Directions:

1. Combine peanut butter, soy sauce, sesame oil, sambal oelek, and water in a bowl.
2. Place the cucumber slices on a dish. Garnish with grated chicken and sprinkle with sauce.
3. Sprinkle the chopped peanuts.

German Hot Potato Salad

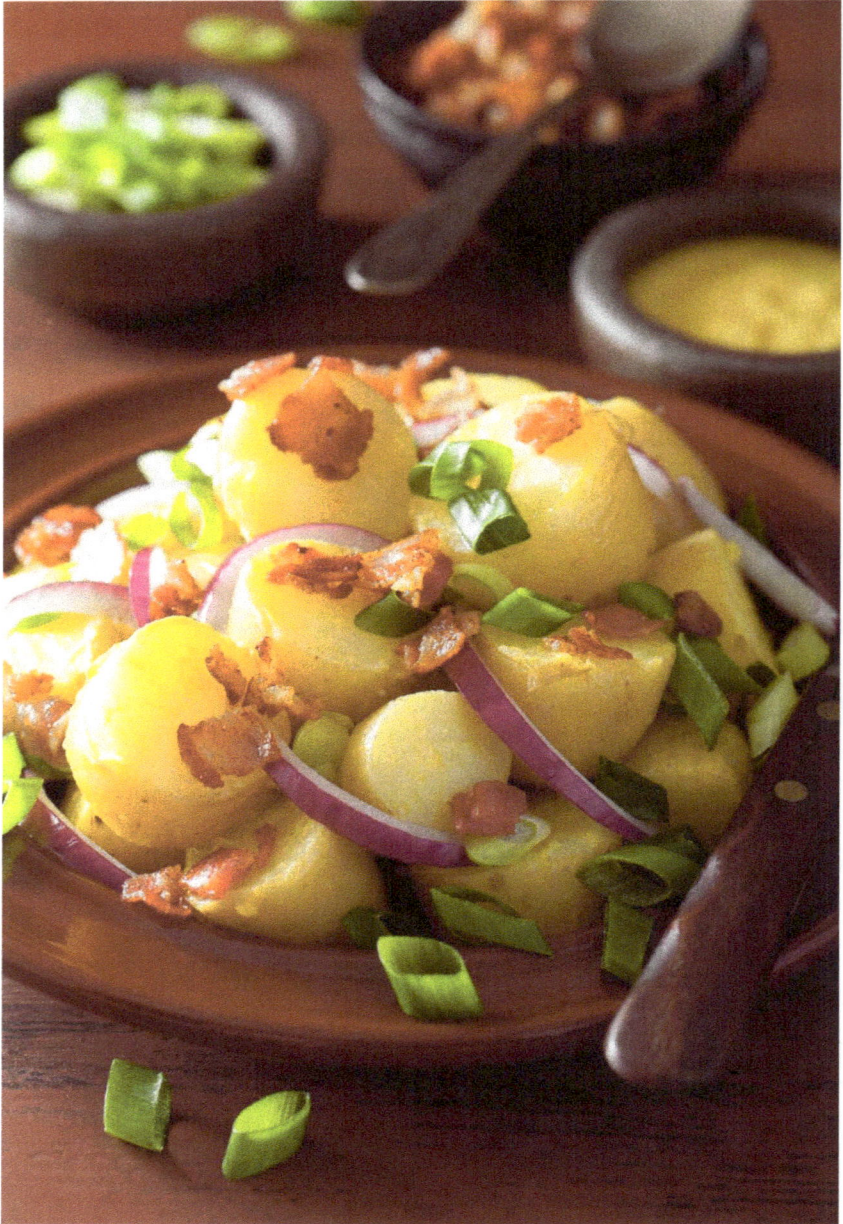

Preparation Time: 10 Minutes
Cooking Time: 30 Minutes
Servings: 12

Nutrition:
Calories:205
Fat:6.5g
Carbohydrates:32.9g
Protein:4.3g
Sodium:814mg
Ingredients:

- 9 peeled potatoes
- 6 slices of bacon
- 1/8 teaspoon ground black pepper
- 1/2 teaspoon celery seed
- 2 tablespoons white sugar
- 2 teaspoons salt
- 3/4 cup water
- 1/3 cup distilled white vinegar
- 2 tablespoons all-purpose flour
- 3/4 cup chopped onions

Directions:

1. Boil salted water in a large pot. Put in the potatoes and cook until soft but still firm, about 30 minutes. Drain, let cool and cut finely.
2. Over medium heat, cook bacon in a pan. Drain, crumble and set aside. Save the cooking juices.
3. Cook onions in bacon grease until golden brown.
4. Combine flour, sugar, salt, celery seed, and pepper in a small bowl. Add sautéed onions and cook, stirring until bubbling, and remove from heat.
5. Stir in the water and vinegar, then bring back to the fire and bring to a boil, stirring constantly. Boil and stir.
6. Slowly add bacon and potato slices to the vinegar/water mixture, stirring gently until the potatoes are warmed up.

Chicken Fiesta Salad

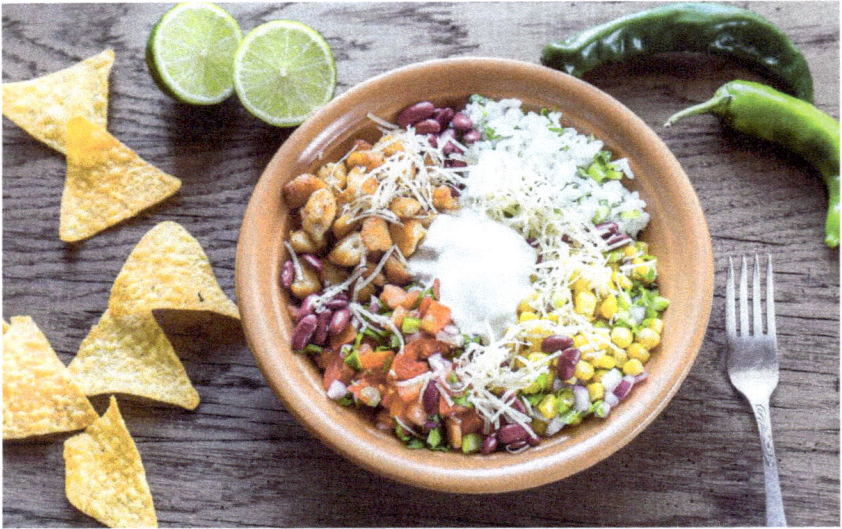

Preparation Time: 20 Minutes
Cooking Time: 20 Minutes
Servings: 4
Nutrition:
Calories:311
Fat:6.4g
Carbohydrates:42.2g
Protein:23g
Sodium:853mg

Ingredients:

- 2 halves of chicken fillet without skin or bones
- 1 packet of herbs for fajitas, divided
- 1 tablespoon vegetable oil
- 1 can black beans, rinsed and drained
- 1 box of Mexican-style corn
- 1/2 cup of salsa
- 1 packet of green salad
- 1 onion, minced
- 1 tomato, quartered

Directions:

1. Rub the chicken evenly with 1/2 of the herbs for fajitas.
2. Cook the oil in a frying pan over medium heat and cook the chicken for 8 minutes on the side by side or until the juice is clear; put aside.
3. Combine beans, corn, salsa, and other 1/2 fajita spices in a large pan.
4. Heat over medium heat until lukewarm.
5. Prepare the salad by mixing green vegetables, onion, and tomato. Cover the chicken salad and dress the beans and corn mixture.

Corn & Black Bean Salad

Preparation Time: 10 Minutes
Cooking Time: 0 Minutes
Servings: 4
Nutrition:
Calories:214
Fat:8.4g
Carbohydrates:28.6g
Protein:7.5g
Sodium:415mg
Ingredients:

- 2 tablespoons vegetable oil
- 1/4 cup balsamic vinegar
- 1/2 teaspoon of salt
- 1/2 teaspoon of white sugar
- 1/2 teaspoon ground cumin
- 1/2 teaspoon ground black pepper
- 1/2 teaspoon chili powder
- 3 tablespoons chopped fresh coriander
- 1 can black beans (15 oz)
- 1 can of sweetened corn (8.75 oz) drained

Directions:

1. Combine balsamic vinegar, oil, salt, sugar, black pepper, cumin and chili powder in a small bowl.

2. Combine black corn and beans in a medium bowl.
3. Mix with vinegar and oil vinaigrette and garnish with coriander. Cover and refrigerate overnight.

Awesome Pasta Salad

Preparation Time: 30 Minutes
Cooking Time: 10 Minutes
Servings: 16
Nutrition:
Calories:310
Fat:17.7g
Carbohydrates:25.9g
Protein:12.9g
Sodium:746mg
Ingredients:

- 1 (16-oz) fusilli pasta package
- 3 cups of cherry tomatoes
- 1/2 pound of provolone, diced
- 1/2 pound of sausage, diced
- 1/4 pound of pepperoni, cut in half
- 1 large green pepper
- 1 can of black olives, drained
- 1 jar of chilis, drained
- 1 bottle (8 oz) Italian vinaigrette

Directions:

1. Boil a lightly salted water in a pot. Stir in the pasta and cook for about 8 to 10 minutes or until al dente. Drain and rinse with cold water.
2. Combine pasta with tomatoes, cheese, salami, pepperoni, green pepper, olives, and peppers in a large bowl. Pour the vinaigrette and mix well.

Southern Potato Salad

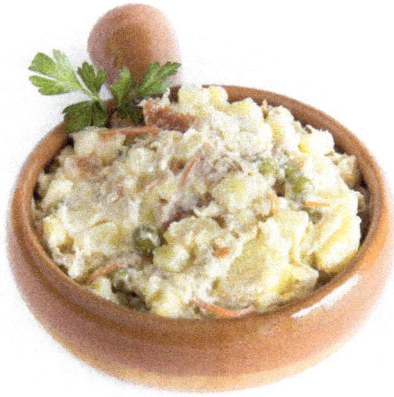

Preparation Time: 15 Minutes
Cooking Time: 15 Minutes
Servings: 4

Nutrition:
Calories:460
Fat:27.4g
Carbohydrates:44.6g
Protein:11.3g
Sodium:214mg
Ingredients:

- 4 potatoes
- 4 eggs
- 1/2 stalk of celery, finely chopped
- 1/4 cup sweet taste
- 1 clove of garlic minced
- 2 tablespoons mustard
- 1/2 cup mayonnaise
- salt and pepper to taste

Directions:

1. Boil water in a pot then situate the potatoes and cook until soft but still firm, about 15 minutes; drain and chop. Transfer the eggs in a pan and cover with cold water.
2. Boil the water; cover, remove from heat, and let the eggs soak in hot water for 10 minutes. Remove then shell and chop.
3. Combine potatoes, eggs, celery, sweet sauce, garlic, mustard, mayonnaise, salt, and pepper in a large bowl. Mix and serve hot.

Seven-Layer Salad

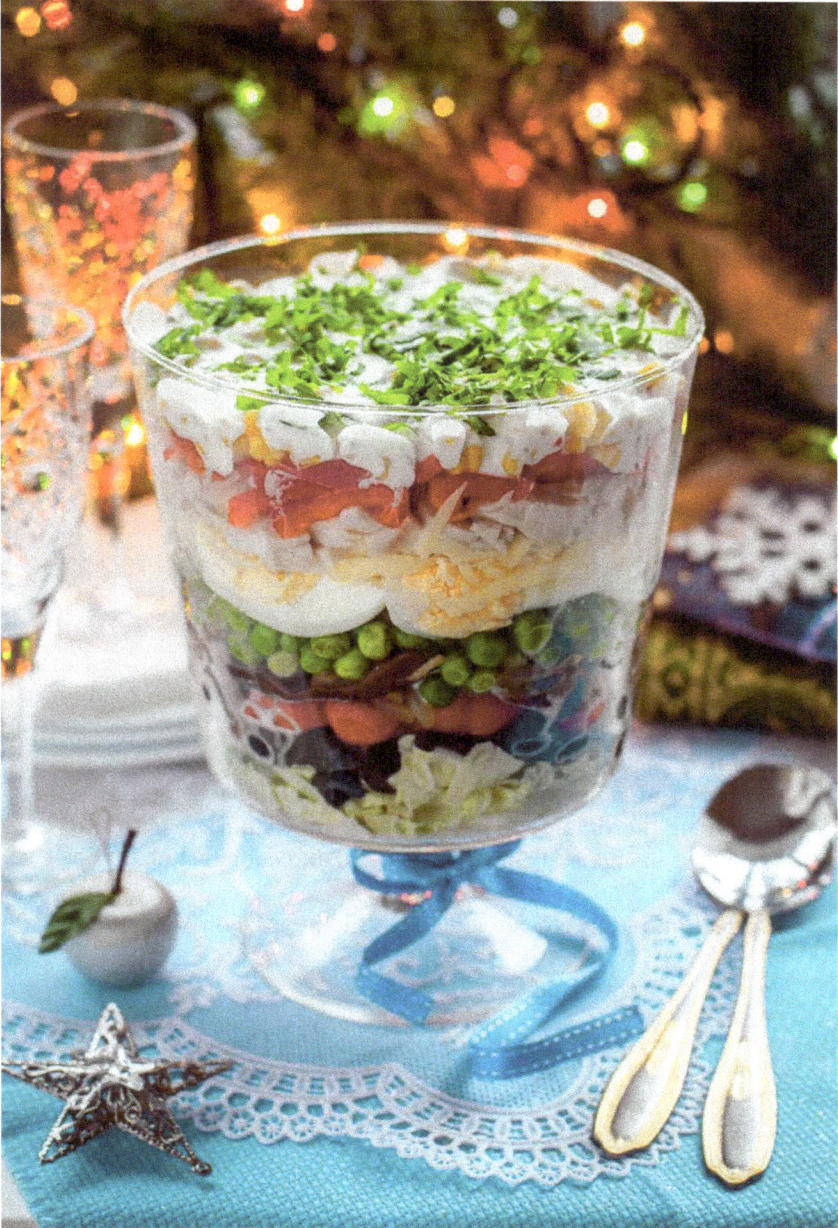

Preparation Time: 15 Minutes
Cooking Time: 5 Minutes
Servings: 10

Nutrition:
Calories:387
Fat:32.7g
Carbohydrates:9.9g
Protein:14.5g
Sodium:609mg
Ingredients:

- 1-pound bacon
- 1 head iceberg lettuce
- 1 red onion, minced
- 1 pack of 10 frozen peas, thawed
- 10 oz grated cheddar cheese
- 1 cup chopped cauliflower
- 1 1/4 cup mayonnaise
- 2 tablespoons white sugar
- 2/3 cup grated Parmesan cheese

Directions:

1. Put the bacon in a huge, shallow frying pan. Bake over medium heat until smooth. Crumble and set aside.
2. Situate the chopped lettuce in a large bowl and cover with a layer of an onion, peas, grated cheese, cauliflower, and bacon.
3. Prepare the vinaigrette by mixing the mayonnaise, sugar, and parmesan cheese. Pour over the salad and cool to cool.

Kale, Quinoa & Avocado Salad with Lemon Dijon Vinaigrette

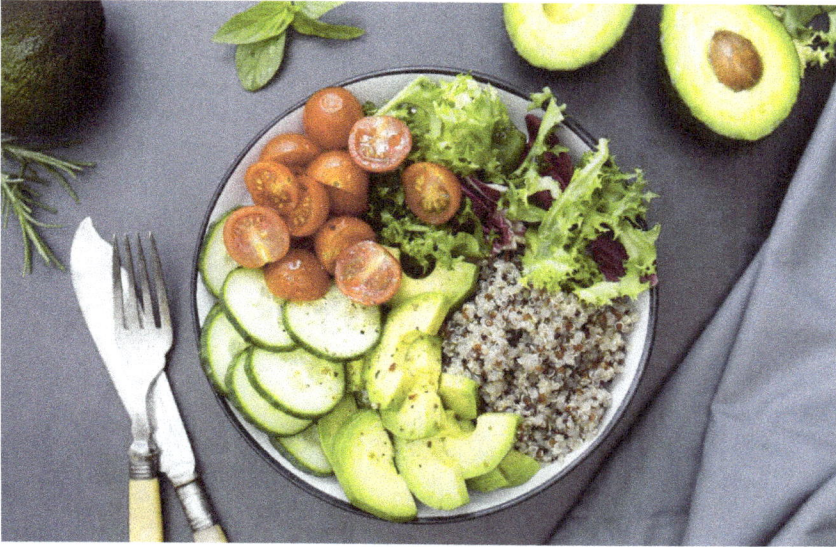

Preparation Time: 5 Minutes
Cooking Time: 25 Minutes
Servings: 4
Nutrition:
Calories:342
Fat:20.3g
Carbohydrates:35.4g
Protein:8.9g
Sodium:705mg
Ingredients:

- 2/3 cup of quinoa
- 1 1/3 cup of water
- 1 bunch of kale
- 1/2 avocado, diced and pitted
- 1/2 cup chopped cucumber
- 1/3 cup chopped red pepper
- 2 tablespoons chopped red onion
- 1 tablespoon of feta crumbled

Directions:

1. Boil the quinoa and 1 1/3 cup of water in a pan. Adjust heat

and simmer until quinoa is tender and water is absorbed for about 15 to 20 minutes. Set aside to cool.

2. Place the cabbage in a steam basket over more than an inch of boiling water in a pan. Seal the pan with a lid and steam until hot, about 45 seconds; transfer to a large plate. Garnish with cabbage, quinoa, avocado, cucumber, pepper, red onion, and feta cheese.

3. Combine olive oil, lemon juice, Dijon mustard, sea salt, and black pepper in a bowl until the oil is emulsified in the dressing; pour over the salad.

Chicken Salad

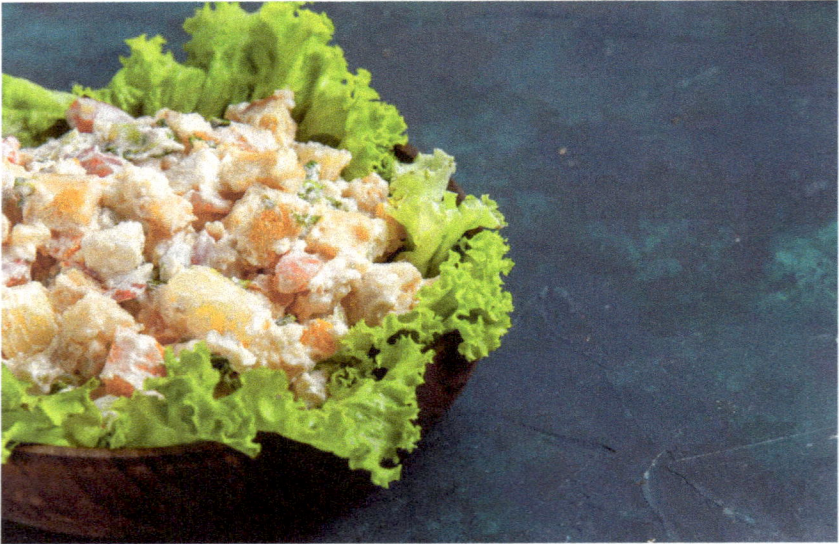

Preparation Time: 20 Minutes
Cooking Time: 0 Minutes
Servings: 9
Nutrition:
Calories:293
Fat:19.5g
Carbohydrates:10.3g
Protein:19.4g
Sodium:454mg

. . .

Ingredients:

- 1/2 cup mayonnaise
- 1/2 teaspoon of salt
- 3/4 teaspoon of poultry herbs
- 1 tablespoon lemon juice
- 3 cups cooked chicken breast, diced
- 1/4 teaspoon ground black pepper
- 1/4 teaspoon garlic powder
- 1/4 teaspoon onion powder
- 1/2 cup finely chopped celery
- 1 (8 oz) box of water chestnuts, drained and chopped
- 1/2 cup chopped green onions
- 1 1/2 cups green grapes cut in half
- 1 1/2 cups diced Swiss cheese

Directions:

1. Combine mayonnaise, salt, chicken spices, onion powder, garlic powder, pepper, and lemon juice in a medium bowl.
2. Combine chicken, celery, green onions, water chestnuts, Swiss cheese, and raisins in a big bowl.
3. Stir in the mayonnaise mixture and coat. Cool until ready to serve.

Cobb Salad

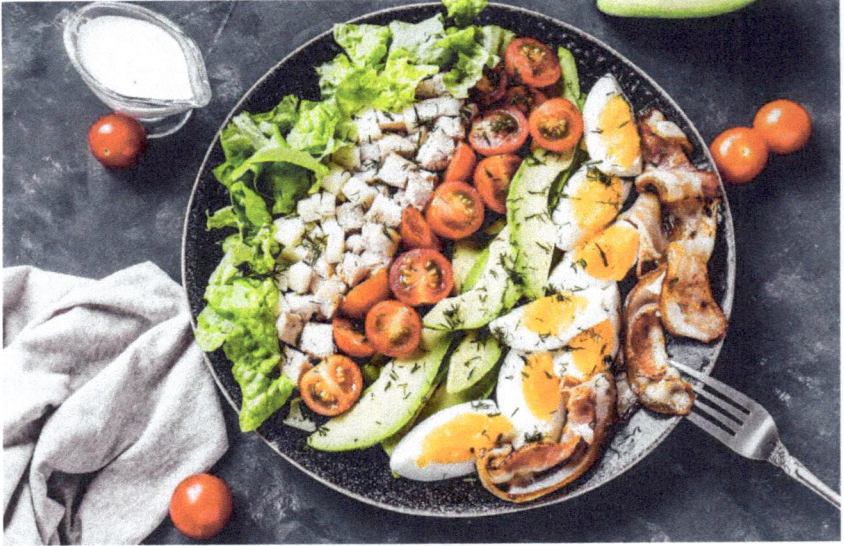

Preparation Time: 5 Minutes
Cooking Time: 15 Minutes
Servings: 6
Nutrition:
Calories:525
Fat:39.9g
Carbohydrates:10.2g
Protein:31.7g
sodium:701mg

Ingredients:

- 6 slices of bacon
- 3 eggs
- 1 cup Iceberg lettuce, grated
- 3 cups cooked minced chicken meat
- 2 tomatoes, seeded and minced
- 3/4 cup of blue cheese, crumbled
- 1 avocado - peeled, pitted and diced
- 3 green onions, minced
- 1 bottle (8 oz.) Ranch Vinaigrette

Directions:

1. Situate the eggs in a pan and soak them completely with cold water. Boil the water. Cover and remove from heat and let the eggs rest in hot water for 10 to 12 minutes. Remove from hot water, let cool, peel, and chop. Situate the bacon in a big, deep frying pan.
2. Bake over medium heat until smooth. Set aside.
3. Divide the grated lettuce into separate plates. Spread chicken, eggs, tomatoes, blue cheese, bacon, avocado, and green onions in rows on lettuce. Sprinkle with your favorite vinaigrette and enjoy.

4

Vegan Recipes

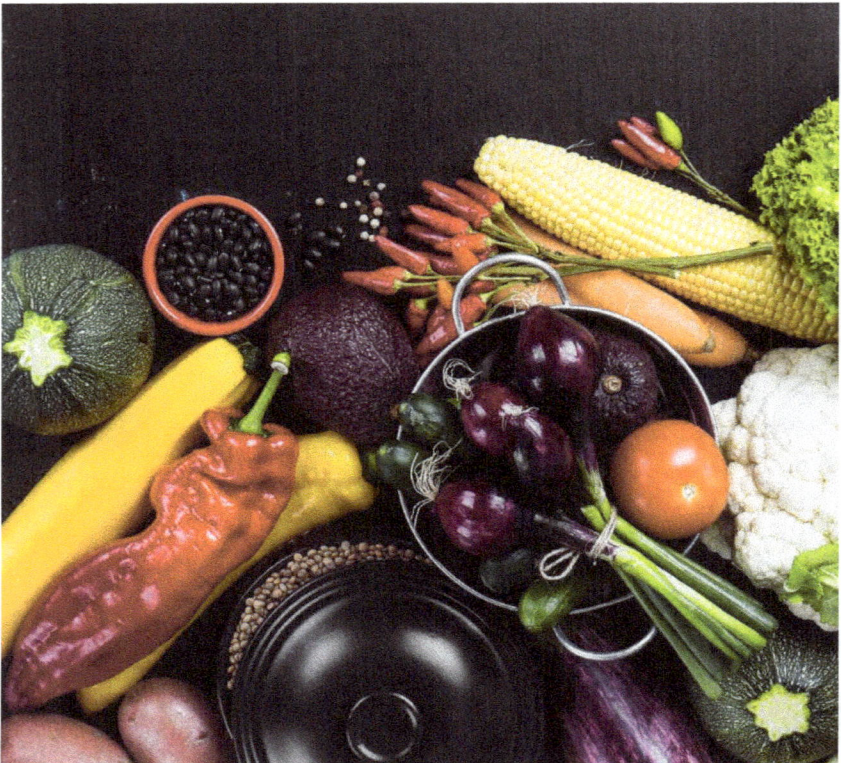

Mediterranean Veggie Bowl

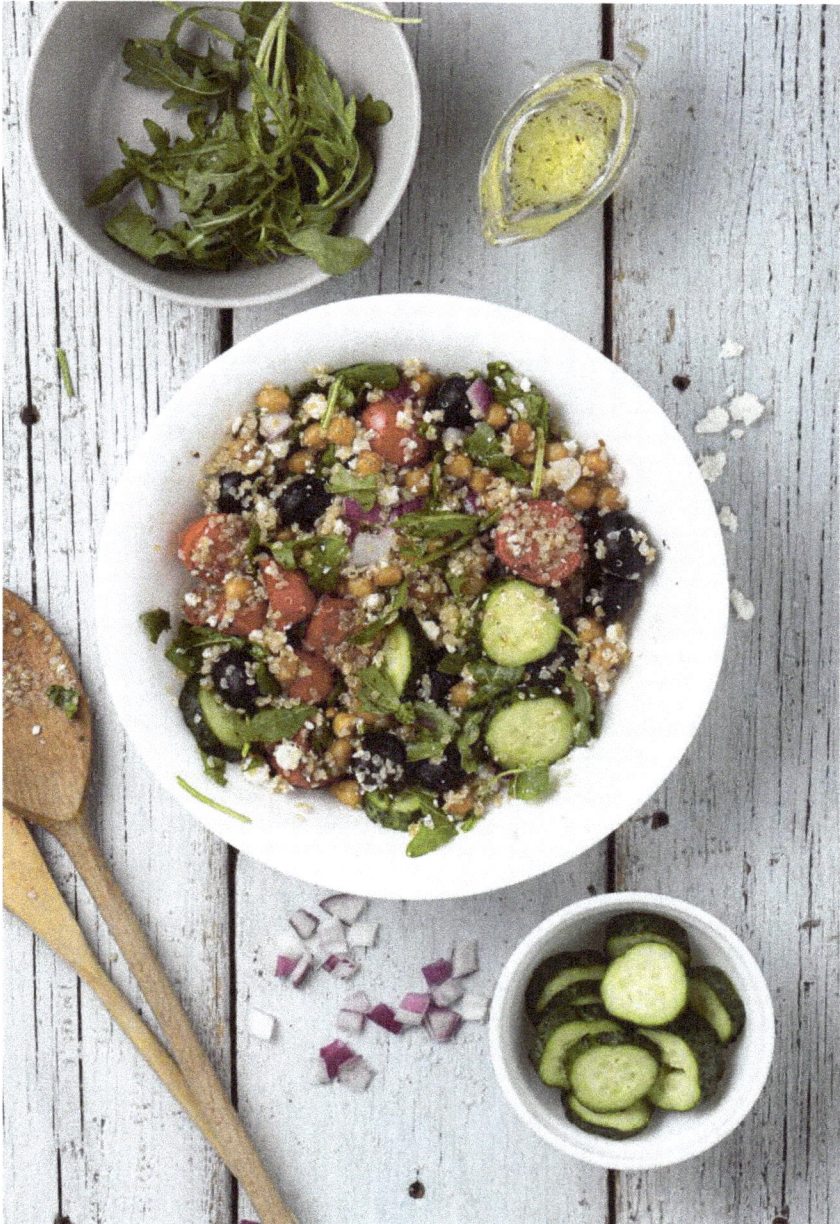

Preparation Time: 10 Minutes

Cooking Time: 20 Minutes
Servings: 4

Nutrition:

Calories: 772
Protein: 6g
Carbohydrates: 41g

Ingredients:

- 1 cup quinoa, rinsed
- 1½ teaspoons salt, divided
- 2 cups cherry tomatoes, cut in half
- 1 large bell pepper, cucumber
- 1 cup Kalamata olives

Directions:

1. Using medium pot over medium heat, boil 2 cups of water. Add the bulgur (or quinoa) and 1 teaspoon of salt. Cover and cook for 15 to 20 minutes.
2. To arrange the veggies in your 4 bowls, visually divide each bowl into 5 sections. Place the cooked bulgur in one section. Follow with the tomatoes, bell pepper, cucumbers, and olives.
3. Scourge ½ cup of lemon juice, olive oil, remaining ½ teaspoon salt, and black pepper.
4. Evenly spoon the dressing over the 4 bowls.
5. Serve immediately or cover and refrigerate for later.

Grilled Veggie and Hummus Wrap

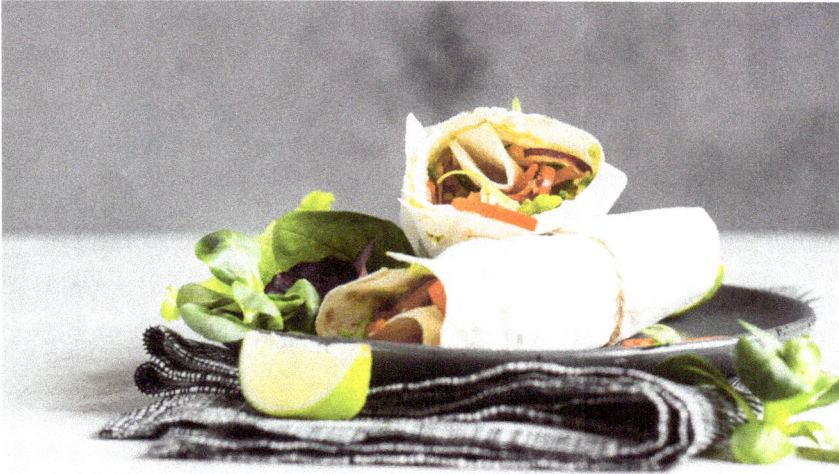

Preparation Time: 15 Minutes
Cooking Time: 10 Minutes
Servings: 6

Nutrition:
Calories: 362
Protein: 15g
Carbohydrates: 28g

Ingredients:

- 1 large eggplant
- 1 large onion
- ½ cup extra-virgin olive oil
- 6 lavash wraps or large pita bread
- 1 cup Creamy Traditional Hummus

Directions:

1. Preheat a grill, large grill pan, or lightly oiled large skillet on medium heat.

2. Slice the eggplant and onion into circles. Rub the vegetables with olive oil and sprinkle with salt.
3. Cook the vegetables on both sides, about 3 to 4 minutes each side.
4. To make the wrap, lay the lavash or pita flat. Spread about 2 tablespoons of hummus on the wrap.
5. Evenly divide the vegetables among the wraps, layering them along one side of the wrap. Gently fold over the side of the wrap with the vegetables, tucking them in and making a tight wrap.
6. Lay the wrap seam side-down and cut in half or thirds.
7. You can also wrap each sandwich with plastic wrap to help it hold its shape and eat it later.

Spanish Green Beans

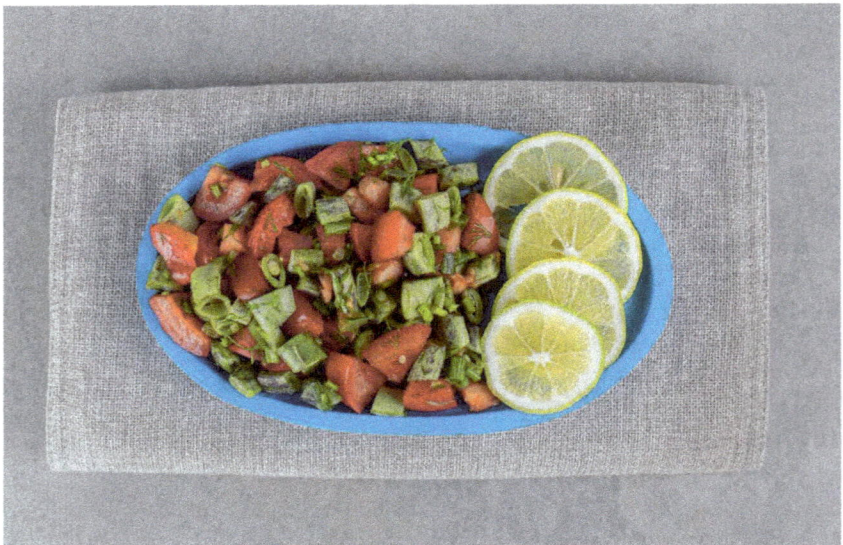

Preparation Time: 10 Minutes
Cooking Time: 20 Minutes
Servings: 4

Nutrition:
Calories: 200
Protein: 4g

Carbohydrates: 18g

Ingredients:

- 1 large onion, chopped
- 4 cloves garlic, finely chopped
- 1-pound green beans, fresh or frozen, trimmed
- 1 (15-ounce) can diced tomatoes

Directions:

1. In a huge pot over medium heat, cook olive oil, onion, and garlic; cook for 1 minute.
2. Cut the green beans into 2-inch pieces.
3. Add the green beans and 1 teaspoon of salt to the pot and toss everything together; cook for 3 minutes.
4. Add the diced tomatoes, remaining ½ teaspoon of salt, and black pepper to the pot; continue to cook for another 12 minutes, stirring occasionally.
5. Serve warm.

Rustic Cauliflower and Carrot Hash

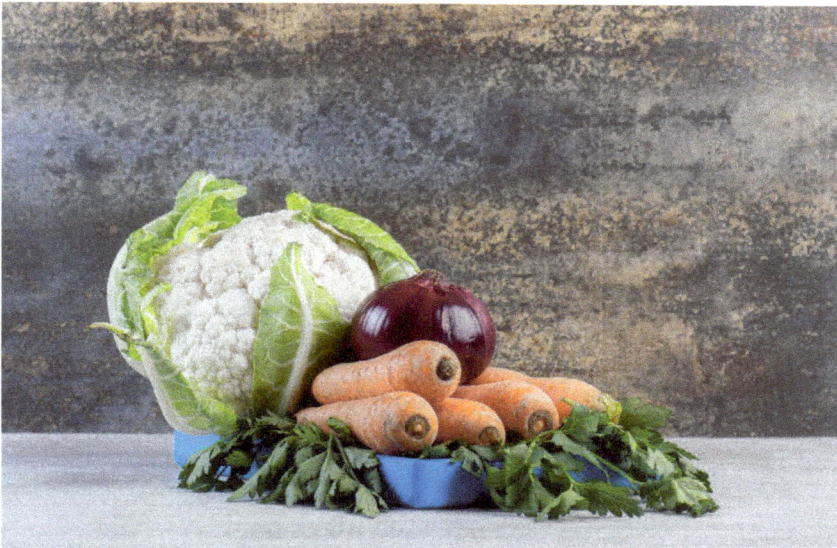

Preparation Time: 10 Minutes
Cooking Time: 10 Minutes
Servings: 4

Nutrition:
Calories: 159
Protein: 3g
Carbohydrates: 15g
Ingredients:

- 1 large onion, chopped
- 1 tablespoon garlic, minced
- 2 cups carrots, diced
- 4 cups cauliflower pieces, washed
- ½ teaspoon ground cumin

Directions:

1. In a big frying pan on medium heat, heat up 3 tbsps. of olive oil, onion, garlic, and carrots for 3 minutes.
2. Cut the cauliflower into 1-inch or bite-size pieces. Add the cauliflower, salt, and cumin to the skillet and toss to combine with the carrots and onions.
3. Cover and cook for 3 minutes.
4. Throw the vegetables and continue to cook uncovered for an additional 3 to 4 minutes.
5. Serve warm.

Roasted Cauliflower and Tomatoes

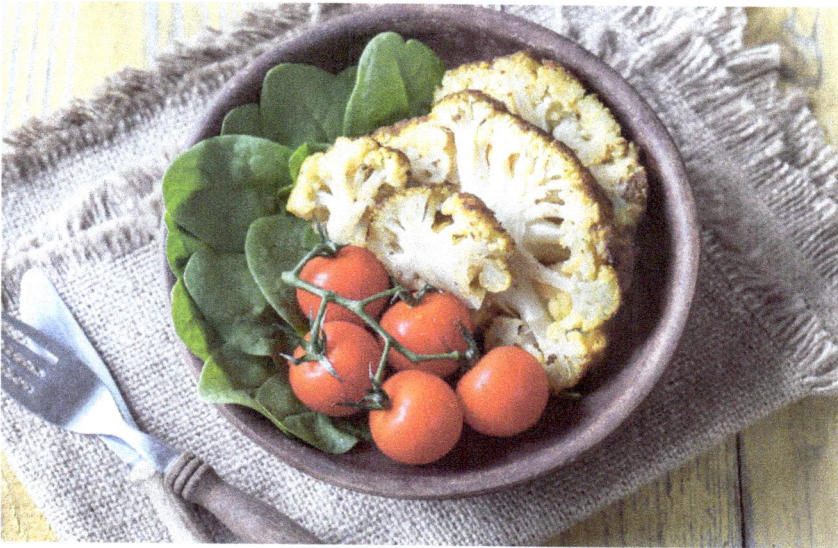

Preparation Time: 5 Minutes
Cooking Time: 25 Minutes
Servings: 4

Nutrition:
Calories: 294
Protein: 9g
Carbohydrates: 13g
Ingredients:

- 4 cups cauliflower, cut into 1-inch pieces
- 6 tablespoons extra-virgin olive oil, divided
- 4 cups cherry tomatoes
- ½ teaspoon freshly ground black pepper
- ½ cup grated Parmesan cheese

Directions:

1. Preheat the oven to 425°F.
2. Add the cauliflower, 3 tablespoons of olive oil, and ½ teaspoon of salt to a large bowl and toss to evenly coat. Pour onto a baking sheet and spread the cauliflower out in an even layer.

3. In another large bowl, add the tomatoes, remaining 3 tablespoons of olive oil, and ½ teaspoon of salt, and toss to coat evenly. Pour onto a different baking sheet.
4. Put the sheet of cauliflower and the sheet of tomatoes in the oven to roast for 17 to 20 minutes until the cauliflower is lightly browned and tomatoes are plump.
5. Using a spatula, spoon the cauliflower into a serving dish, and top with tomatoes, black pepper, and Parmesan cheese. Serve warm.

Roasted Acorn Squash

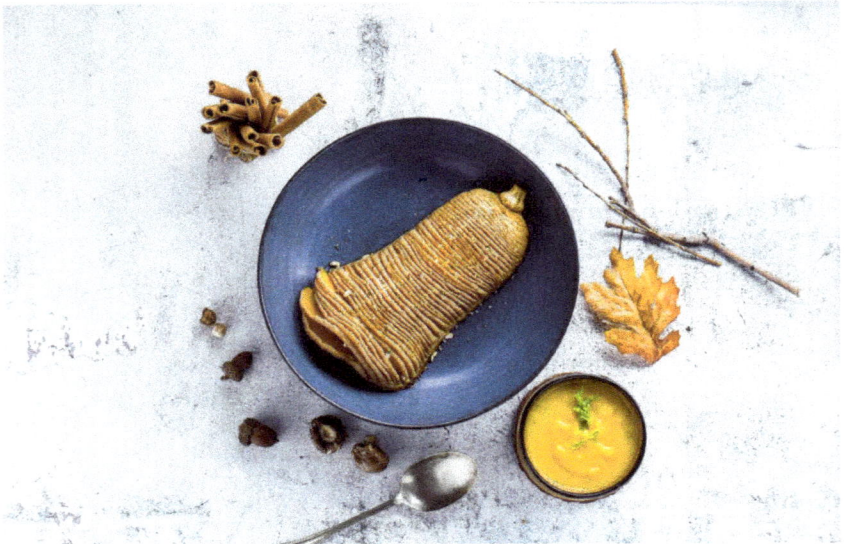

Preparation Time: 10 Minutes
Cooking Time: 35 Minutes
Servings: 6

Nutrition:
Calories: 188
Protein: 1g
Carbohydrates: 16g

Ingredients:

- 2 acorn squash, medium to large
- 2 tablespoons extra-virgin olive oil
- 5 tablespoons unsalted butter
- ¼ cup chopped sage leaves
- 2 tablespoons fresh thyme leaves

Directions:

1. Preheat the oven to 400°F.
2. Cut the acorn squash in half lengthwise. Scoop out the seeds and cut it horizontally into ¾-inch-thick slices.
3. In a large bowl, drizzle the squash with the olive oil, sprinkle with salt, and toss together to coat.
4. Lay the acorn squash flat on a baking sheet.
5. Put the baking sheet in the oven and bake the squash for 20 minutes. Flip squash over with a spatula and bake for another 15 minutes.
6. Melt the butter in a medium saucepan over medium heat.
7. Add the sage and thyme to the melted butter and let them cook for 30 seconds.
8. Transfer the cooked squash slices to a plate. Spoon the butter/herb mixture over the squash. Season with salt and black pepper. Serve warm.

Sautéed Garlic Spinach

Preparation Time: 5 Minutes
Cooking Time: 10 Minutes
Servings: 4
Nutrition:
Calories: 301
Protein: 17g
Carbohydrates: 29g
Ingredients:

- ¼ cup extra-virgin olive oil
- 1 large onion, thinly sliced
- 3 cloves garlic, minced
- 6 (1-pound) bags of baby spinach, washed

- 1 lemon, cut into wedges

Directions:

1. Cook the olive oil, onion, and garlic in a large skillet for 2 minutes over medium heat.
2. Add one bag of spinach and ½ teaspoon of salt. Cover the skillet and let the spinach wilt for 30 seconds. Repeat (omitting the salt), adding 1 bag of spinach at a time.
3. Once all the spinach has been added, remove the cover and cook for 3 minutes, letting some of the moisture evaporate.
4. Serve warm with lemon juice over the top.

Garlicky Sautéed Zucchini with Mint

Preparation Time: 5 Minutes
Cooking Time: 10 Minutes
Servings: 4
Nutrition:
Calories: 147
Protein: 4g
Carbohydrates: 12g
Ingredients:

- 3 large green zucchinis
- 3 tablespoons extra-virgin olive oil
- 1 large onion, chopped
- 3 cloves garlic, minced
- 1 teaspoon dried mint

Directions:

1. Cut the zucchini into ½-inch cubes.
2. Using huge skillet, place over medium heat, cook the olive oil, onions, and garlic for 3 minutes, stirring constantly.
3. Add the zucchini and salt to the skillet and toss to combine with the onions and garlic, cooking for 5 minutes.
4. Add the mint to the skillet, tossing to combine. Cook for another 2 minutes. Serve warm.

Stewed Okra

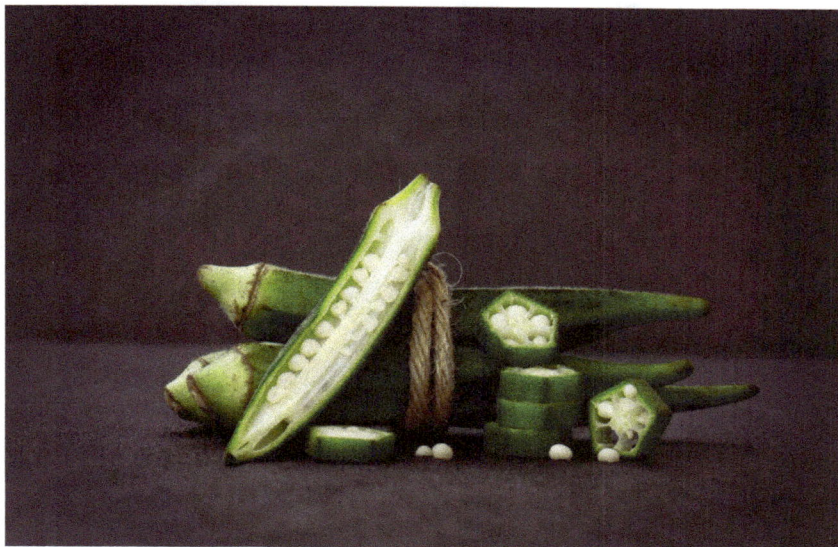

Preparation Time: 5 Minutes
Cooking Time: 25 Minutes
Servings: 4

Nutrition:
Calories: 201
Protein: 4g
Carbohydrates: 18g

Ingredients:

- 4 cloves garlic, finely chopped
- 1 pound fresh or frozen okra, cleaned
- 1 (15-ounce) can plain tomato sauce
- 2 cups water
- ½ cup fresh cilantro, finely chopped

Directions:

1. In a big pot at medium heat, stir and cook ¼ cup of olive oil, 1 onion, garlic, and salt for 1 minute.

2. Stir in the okra and cook for 3 minutes.
3. Add the tomato sauce, water, cilantro, and black pepper; stir, cover, and let cook for 15 minutes, stirring occasionally.
4. Serve warm.

Sweet Veggie-Stuffed Peppers

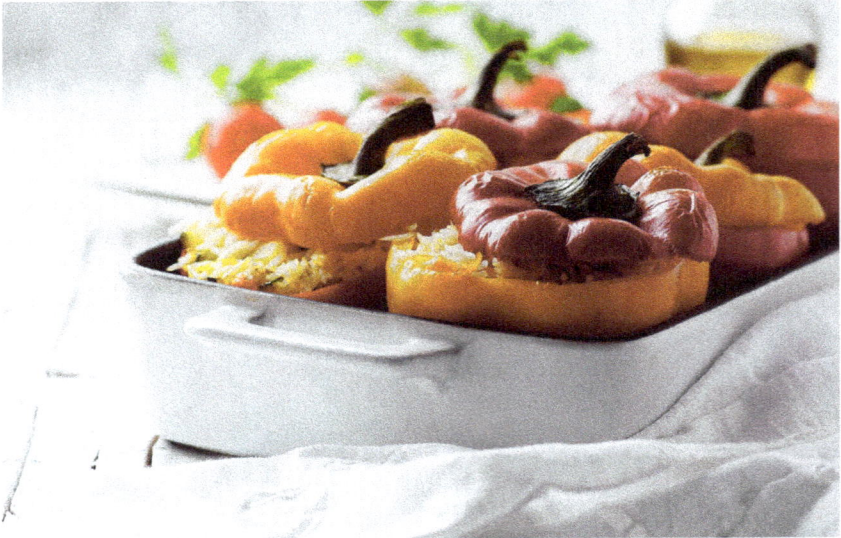

Preparation Time: 20 Minutes
Cooking Time: 30 Minutes
Servings: 6

Nutrition:
Calories: 301
Protein: 8g
Carbohydrates: 50g

Ingredients:

- 6 large bell peppers, different colors
- 3 cloves garlic, minced
- 1 carrot, chopped

- 1 (16-ounce) can garbanzo beans
- 3 cups cooked rice

Directions:

1. **Preheat the oven to 350°F.**
2. **Make sure to choose peppers that can stand upright. Cut off the pepper cap and remove the seeds, reserving the cap for later. Stand the peppers in a baking dish.**
3. **In a skillet over medium heat, cook up olive oil, 1 onion, garlic, and carrots for 3 minutes.**
4. **Stir in the garbanzo beans. Cook for another 3 minutes.**
5. **Remove the pan from the heat and spoon the cooked ingredients to a large bowl.**
6. **Add the rice, salt, and pepper; toss to combine.**
7. **Stuff each pepper to the top and then put the pepper caps back on.**
8. **Cover the baking dish with aluminum foil and bake for 25 minutes.**
9. **Remove the foil and bake for another 5 minutes.**
10. **Serve warm.**

Vegetable-Stuffed Grape Leaves

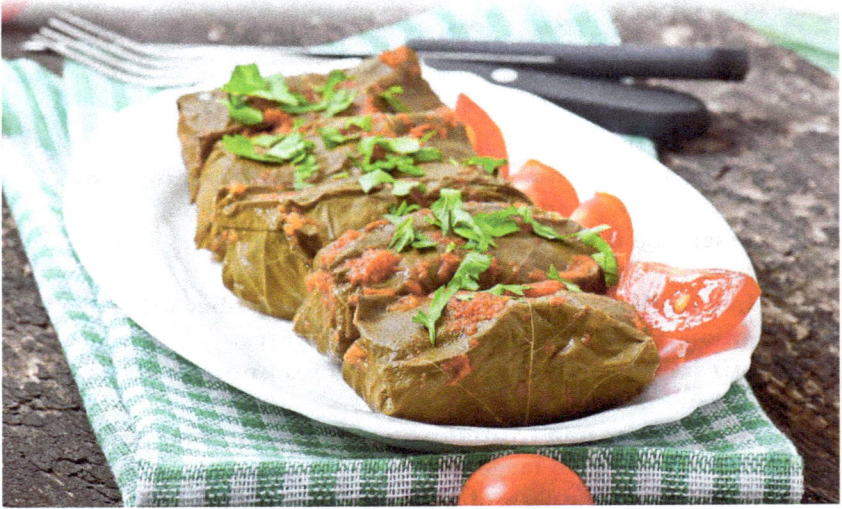

Preparation Time: 50 Minutes
Cooking Time: 45 Minutes
Servings: 7

Nutrition:
Calories: 532
Protein: 12g
Carbohydrates: 80g

Ingredients:

- 2 cups white rice, rinsed
- 2 large tomatoes, finely diced
- 1 (16-ounce) jar grape leaves
- 1 cup lemon juice
- 4 to 6 cups water

Directions:

1. **Incorporate rice, tomatoes, 1 onion, 1 green onion, 1 cup of parsley, 3 garlic cloves, salt, and black pepper.**

2. **Drain and rinse the grape leaves.**
3. **Prepare a large pot by placing a layer of grape leaves on the bottom. Lay each leaf flat and trim off any stems.**
4. **Place 2 tablespoons of the rice mixture at the base of each leaf. Fold over the sides, then roll as tight as possible. Place the rolled grape leaves in the pot, lining up each rolled grape leaf. Continue to layer in the rolled grape leaves.**
5. **Gently pour the lemon juice and olive oil over the grape leaves, and add enough water to just cover the grape leaves by 1 inch.**
6. **Lay a heavy plate that is smaller than the opening of the pot upside down over the grape leaves. Cover the pot and cook the leaves over medium-low heat for 45 minutes. Let stand for 20 minutes before serving.**
7. **Serve warm or cold.**

Grilled Eggplant Rolls

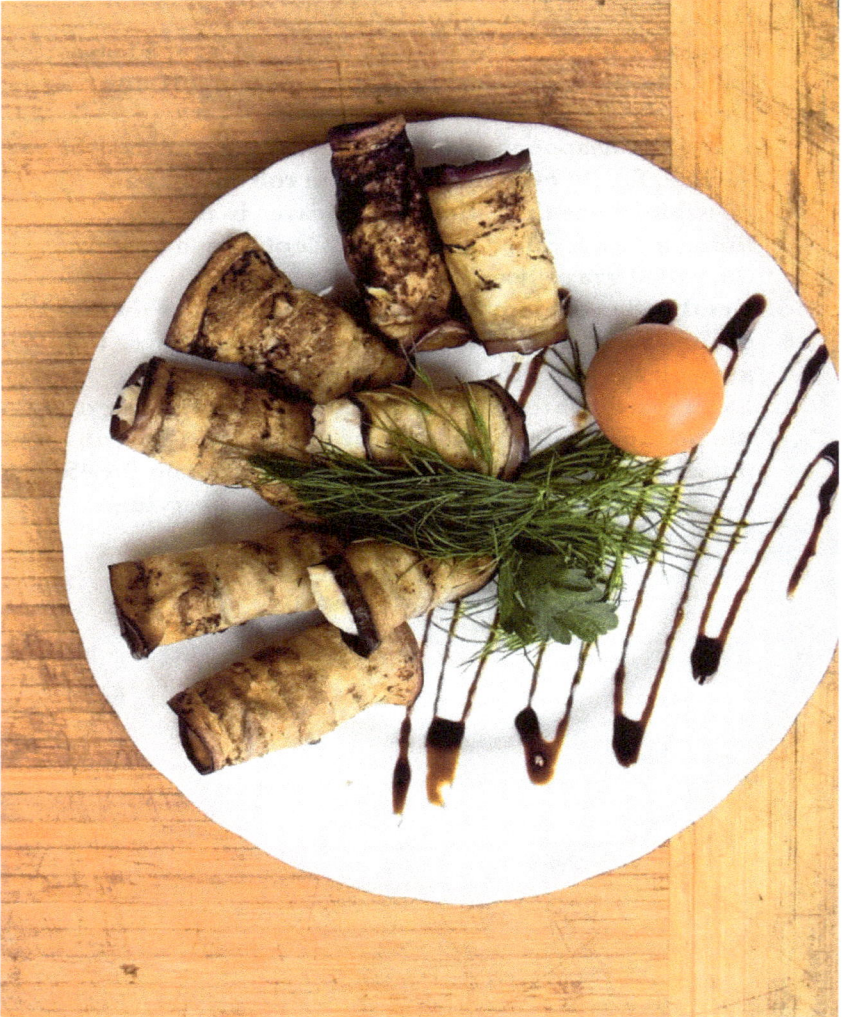

Preparation Time: 30 Minutes
Cooking Time: 10 Minutes
Servings: 5

Nutrition:
Calories: 255
Protein: 15g
Carbohydrates: 19g

. . .

Ingredients:

- 2 large eggplants
- 4 ounces goat cheese
- 1 cup ricotta
- ¼ cup fresh basil, finely chopped

Directions:

1. **Slice the tops of the eggplants off and cut the eggplants lengthwise into ¼-inch-thick slices. Sprinkle the slices with the salt and place the eggplant in a colander for 15 to 20 minutes. The salt will draw out excess water from the eggplant.**
2. **In a large bowl, combine the goat cheese, ricotta, basil, and pepper.**
3. **Preheat a grill, grill pan, or lightly oiled skillet on medium heat. Pat the eggplant slices dry using paper towel and lightly spray with olive oil spray. Place the eggplant on the grill, grill pan, or skillet and cook for 3 minutes on each side.**
4. **Remove the eggplant from the heat and let cool for 5 minutes.**
5. **To roll, lay one eggplant slice flat, place a tablespoon of the cheese mixture at the base of the slice, and roll up. Serve immediately or chill until serving.**

Crispy Zucchini Fritters

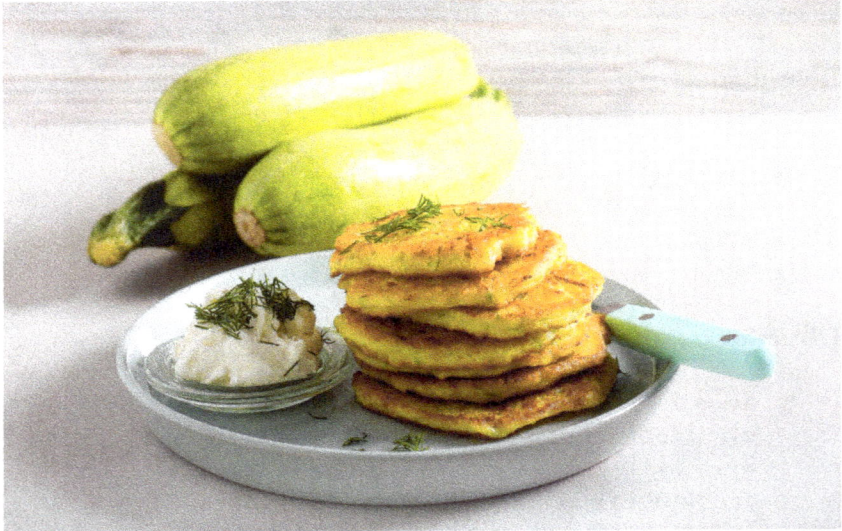

Preparation Time: 15 Minutes
Cooking Time: 20 Minutes
Servings: 6

Nutrition:
Calories: 446
Protein: 5g
Carbohydrates: 19g

Ingredients:

- 2 large green zucchinis
- 1 cup flour
- 1 large egg, beaten
- ½ cup water
- 1 teaspoon baking powder

Directions:

1. **Grate the zucchini into a large bowl.**
2. **Add the 2 tbsps. of parsley, 3 garlic cloves, salt, flour,**

egg, water, and baking powder to the bowl and stir to combine.

3. In a large pot or fryer over medium heat, heat oil to 365°F.
4. Drop the fritter batter into 3 cups of vegetable oil. Turn the fritters over using a slotted spoon and fry until they are golden brown, about 2 to 3 minutes.
5. Strain fritters from the oil and place on a plate lined with paper towels.
6. Serve warm with Creamy Tzatziki or Creamy Traditional Hummus as a dip.

Cheesy Spinach Pies

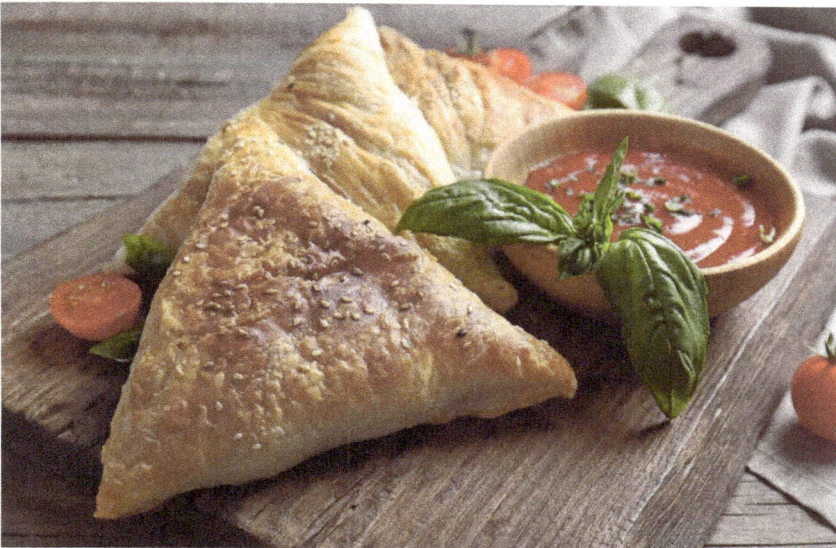

Preparation Time: 20 Minutes
Cooking Time: 40 Minutes
Servings: 5

Nutrition:
Calories: 503
Protein: 16g
Carbohydrates: 38g

. . .

Ingredients:

- 2 tablespoons extra-virgin olive oil
- 3 (1-pound) bags of baby spinach, washed
- 1 cup feta cheese
- 1 large egg, beaten
- Puff pastry sheets

Directions:

1. **Preheat the oven to 375°F.**
2. **In a frying pan on medium heat, put the olive oil, 1 onion, and 2 garlic cloves for 3 minutes.**
3. **Add the spinach to the skillet one bag at a time, letting it wilt in between each bag. Toss using tongs. Cook for 4 minutes. Once the spinach is cooked, drain any excess liquid from the pan.**
4. **Mix feta cheese, egg, and cooked spinach.**
5. **Lay the puff pastry flat on a counter. Cut the pastry into 3-inch squares.**
6. **Place a tablespoon of the spinach mixture in the center of a puff-pastry square. Fold over one corner of the square to the diagonal corner, forming a triangle. Crimp the edges of the pie by pressing down with the tines of a fork to seal them together. Repeat until all squares are filled.**
7. **Situate the pies on a parchment-lined baking sheet and bake for 25 to 30 minutes or until golden brown. Serve warm or at room temperature.**

Instant Pot Black Eyed Peas

Preparation Time: 6 Minutes
Cooking Time: 25 Minutes
Servings: 4
Nutrition:
Calories: 506
Protein: 14g
Carbohydrates: 33g
Ingredients:

- 2 cups black-eyed peas (dried)
- 1 cup parsley, dill
- 2 slices oranges, 2 tbsp. tomato paste
- 4 green onions
- 2 carrots, bay leaves

Directions:

1. **Clean the dill thoroughly with water removing stones.**
2. **Add all the ingredients in the instant pot and stir well to combine.**
3. **Lid the instant pot and set the vent to sealing.**
4. **Set time for twenty-five minutes. When the time has elapsed release pressure naturally.**

Green Beans and Potatoes in Olive Oil

Preparation Time: 12 Minutes
Cooking Time: 17 Minutes
Servings: 4
Nutrition:
Calories: 510
Protein: 20g
Carbohydrates: 28g
Ingredients:

- 15 oz. tomatoes (diced)
- 2 potatoes
- 1 lb. green beans (fresh)
- 1 bunch dill, parsley, zucchini
- 1 tbsp. dried oregano

Directions:

1. **Turn on the sauté function on your instant pot.**
2. **Pour tomatoes, a cup of water and olive oil. Add the rest of the ingredients and stir through.**

3. **Lid the instant pot and set the valve to seal. Set time for fifteen minutes.**
4. **When the time has elapsed release pressure. Remove the Fasolakia from the instant pot. Serve and enjoy.**

Nutritious Vegan Cabbage

Preparation Time: 35 Minutes
Cooking Time: 15 Minutes
Servings: 6
Nutrition:
Calories: 67
Fat: 0.4g
Fiber: 3.8g
Ingredients:

- 3 cups green cabbage
- 1 can tomatoes, onion
- Cups vegetable broth
- 3 stalks celery, carrots
- 2 tbsp. vinegar, sage

Directions:

1. **Mix 1 tbsp. of lemon juice. 2 garlic cloves and the rest of ingredients in the instant pot and. Lid and set time for fifteen minutes on high pressure.**
2. **Release pressure naturally then remove the lid. Remove the soup from the instant pot.**
3. **Serve and enjoy.**

Instant Pot Horta and Potatoes

Preparation Time: 12 Minutes
Cooking Time: 17 Minutes
Servings: 4
Nutrition:
Calories: 499
Protein: 18g

Carbohydrates: 41g
Ingredients:

- 2 heads of washed and chopped greens (spinach, Dandelion, kale, mustard green, Swiss chard)
- 6 potatoes (washed and cut in pieces)
- 1 cup virgin olive oil
- 1 lemon juice (reserve slices for serving)
- 10 garlic cloves (chopped)

Directions:

1. **Position all the ingredients in the instant pot and lid setting the vent to sealing.**
2. **Set time for fifteen minutes. When time is done release pressure.**
3. **Let the potatoes rest for some time. Serve and enjoy with lemon slices.**

Instant Pot Jackfruit Curry

Preparation Time: 1 Hour
Cooking Time: 16 Minutes
Servings: 2
Nutrition:
Calories: 369
Fat: 3g
Fiber: 6g
Ingredients:

- 1 tbsp. oil
- Cumin seeds, Mustard seeds
- 2 tomatoes (purred)
- 20 oz. can green jackfruit (drained and rinsed)
- 1 tbsp. coriander powder, turmeric.

Directions:

1. **Turn the instant pot to sauté mode. Add cumin plus mustard seeds, then allow them to sizzle.**

2. **Add other ingredients, and a cup of water then lid the instant pot. Set time for seven minutes on high pressure.**
3. **When the time has elapsed release pressure naturally, shred the jackfruit and serve.**

Instant Pot Collard Greens with Tomatoes

Preparation Time: 18 Minutes
Cooking Time: 8 Minutes
Servings: 4
Nutrition:
Calories: 498
Protein: 19g
Carbohydrates: 32g
Ingredients:

- 1 white onion (diced)
- 3tbsp olive oil
- 3 garlic cloves (minced)
- Cup tomatoes (sun-dried and chopped)
- 1 bunch collard greens (roughly cut and hard stems removed)

Directions:

1. **Turn on the sauté function on your instant pot.**
2. **Add onions and olive oil to the instant pot and let cook for three minutes or until lightly browned.**
3. **Add the rest of ingredients one at a time while stirring.**
4. **Add salt and pepper to taste and a cup of water. Turn off the sauté function and set to manual. Set time for five minutes at high pressure.**
5. **When the time has elapsed, release pressure naturally.**
6. **Open the lid and drizzle a half lemon juice.**
7. **Serve and enjoy.**

Starters and Sides

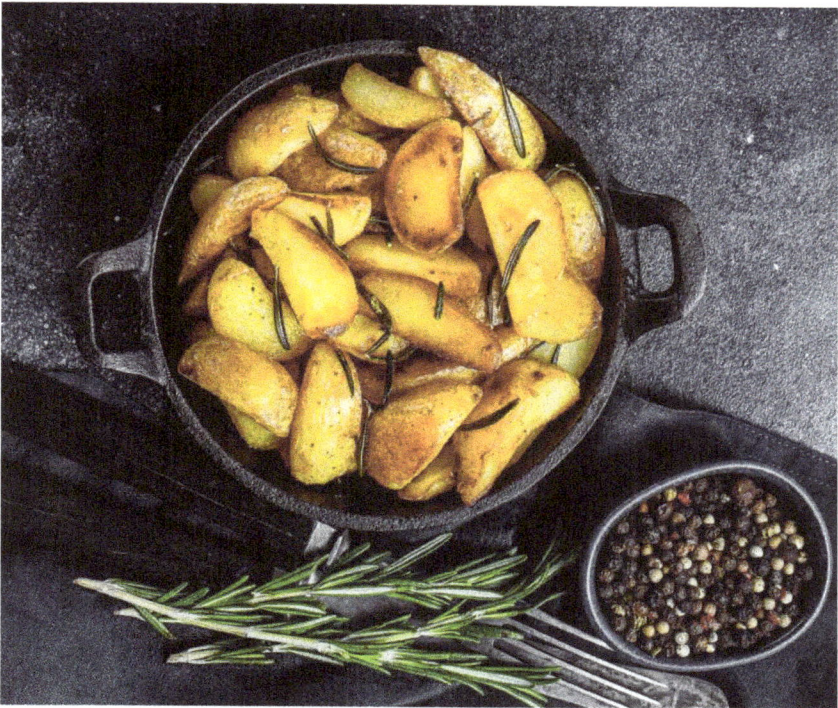

Nachos

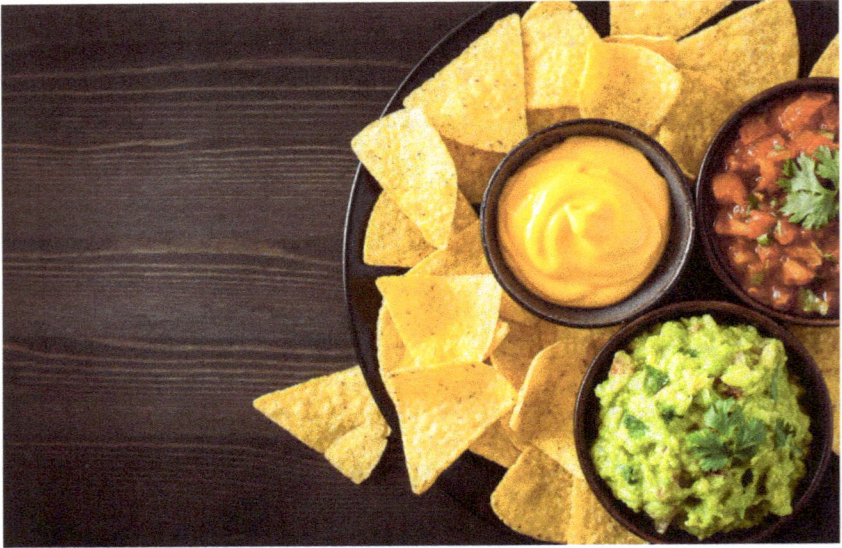

Preparation Time: 5 Minutes
Cooking Time: 10 Minutes
Servings: 4

Nutrition:
Calories: 140
Carbs: 19g
Fat: 7g
Protein: 2g

Ingredients:

- 4-ounce restaurant-style corn tortilla chips
- 1 medium green onion, thinly sliced (about 1 tbsp.)
- 1 (4 ounces) package finely crumbled feta cheese
- 1 finely chopped and drained plum tomato
- 2 tbsp Sun-dried tomatoes in oil, finely chopped
- 2 tbsp Kalamata olives

Directions:

1. Mix an onion, plum tomato, oil, sun-dried tomatoes, and olives in a small bowl.
2. Arrange the tortillas chips on a microwavable plate in a single layer topped evenly with cheese—microwave on high for one minute.
3. Rotate the plate half turn and continue microwaving until the cheese is bubbly. Spread the tomato mixture over the chips and cheese and enjoy.

Stuffed Celery

Preparation Time: 15 Minutes
Cooking Time: 20 Minutes
Servings: 3
Nutrition:
Calories: 64
Carbs: 2g
Fat: 6g
Protein: 1g
Ingredients:

- Olive oil
- 1 clove garlic, minced
- 2 tbsp Pine nuts
- 2 tbsp dry-roasted sunflower seeds
- ¼ cup Italian cheese blend, shredded
- 8 stalks celery leaves
- 1 (8-ounce) fat-free cream cheese
- Cooking spray

Directions:

1. Sauté garlic and pine nuts over a medium setting for the heat until the nuts are golden brown. Cut off the wide base and tops from celery.
2. Remove two thin strips from the round side of the celery to create a flat surface.
3. Mix Italian cheese and cream cheese in a bowl and spread into cut celery stalks.
4. Sprinkle half of the celery pieces with sunflower seeds and a

half with the pine nut mixture. Cover mixture and let stand for at least 4 hours before eating.

Butternut Squash Fries

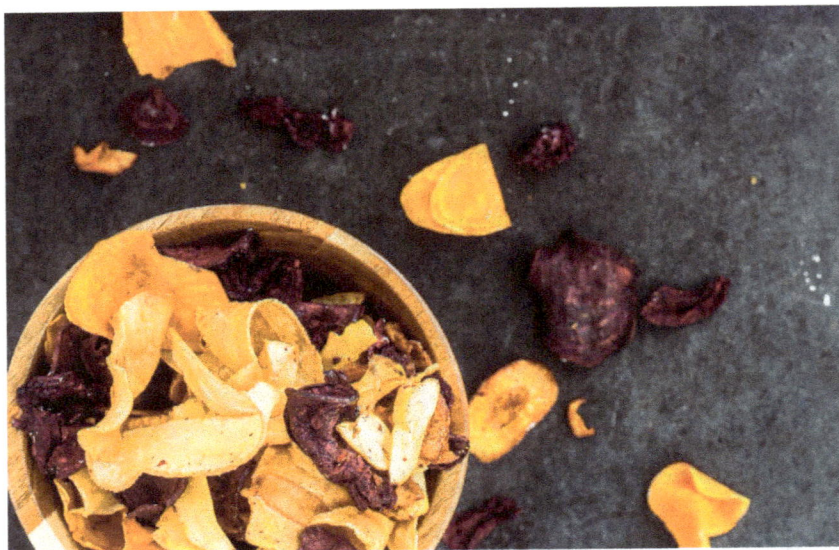

Preparation Time: 5 Minutes
Cooking Time: 10 Minutes
Servings: 2

Nutrition:
Calories: 40
Carbs: 10g
Fat: 0g
Protein: 1g

Ingredients:

- 1 Butternut squash
- 1 tbsp Extra virgin olive oil
- ½ tbsp Grapeseed oil
- 1/8 tsp Sea salt

Directions:

1. Remove seeds from the squash and cut into thin slices. Coat with extra virgin olive oil and grapeseed oil. Add a sprinkle of salt and toss to coat well.
2. Arrange the squash slices onto three baking sheets and bake for 10 minutes until crispy.

Dried Fig Tapenade

Preparation Time: 5 Minutes
Cooking Time: 0 Minutes
Servings: 1
Nutrition:
Calories: 249
Carbs: 64g
Fat: 1g
Protein: 3g
Ingredients:

- 1 cup Dried figs
- 1 cup Kalamata olives
- ½ cup Water
- 1 tbsp Chopped fresh thyme
- 1 tbsp extra virgin olive oil
- ½ tsp Balsamic vinegar

Directions:

1. Prepare figs in a food processor until well chopped, add water, and continue processing to form a paste.
2. Add olives and pulse until well blended. Add thyme, vinegar, and extra virgin olive oil and pulse until very smooth. Best served with crackers of your choice.

Speedy Sweet Potato Chips

Preparation Time: 15 Minutes
Cooking Time: 0 Minutes
Servings: 4
Nutrition:

Calories: 150
Carbs: 16g
Fat: 9g
Protein: 1g
Ingredients:

- 1 large Sweet potato
- 1 tbsp Extra virgin olive oil
- Salt

Directions:

1. 300°F preheated oven. Slice your potato into nice, thin slices that resemble fries.
2. Toss the potato slices with salt and extra virgin olive oil in a bowl. Bake for about one hour, flipping every 15 minutes until crispy and browned.

Nachos with Hummus (Mediterranean Inspired)

Preparation Time: 15 Minutes
Cooking Time: 20 Minutes
Servings: 4
Nutrition:
Calories: 130
Carbs: 18g
Fat: 5g
Protein: 4g
Ingredients:

- 4 cups salted pita chips
- 1 (8 oz.) red pepper (roasted)
- Hummus
- 1 tsp Finely shredded lemon peel
- ¼ cup Chopped pitted Kalamata olives
- ¼ cup crumbled feta cheese
- 1 plum (Roma) tomato, seeded, chopped
- ½ cup chopped cucumber
- 1 tsp Chopped fresh oregano leaves

Directions:

1. 400°F preheated oven. Arrange the pita chips on a heatproof platter and drizzle with hummus.
2. Top with olives, tomato, cucumber, and cheese and bake until warmed through. Sprinkle lemon zest and oregano and enjoy while it's hot.

Hummus and Olive Pita Bread

Preparation Time: 5 Minutes
Cooking Time: 0 Minutes
Servings: 3
Nutrition:
Calories: 225
Carbs: 40g
Fat: 5g
Protein: 9g
Ingredients:

- 7 pita bread cut into 6 wedges each
- 1 (7 ounces) container plain hummus
- 1 tbsp Greek vinaigrette
- ½ cup Chopped pitted Kalamata olives

Directions:

1. Spread the hummus on a serving plate—Mix vinaigrette and olives in a bowl and spoon over the hummus. Enjoy with wedges of pita bread.

Roast Asparagus

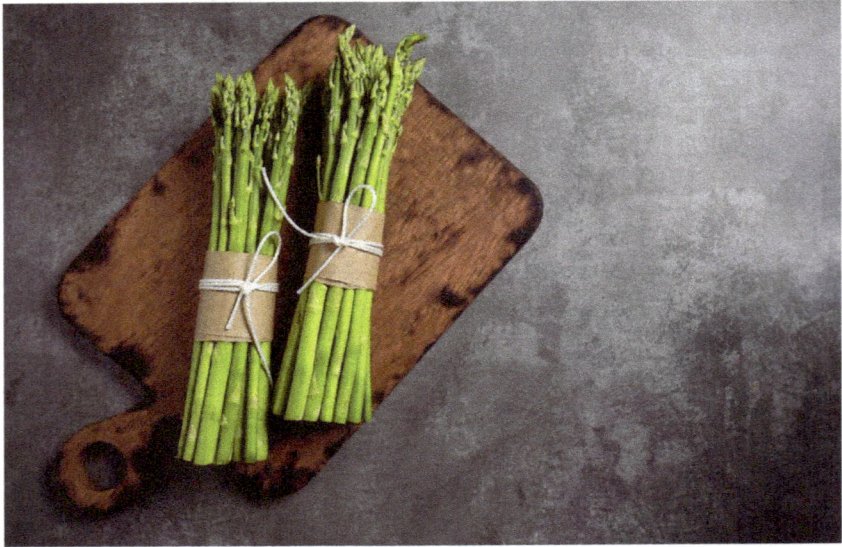

Preparation Time: 15 Minutes
Cooking Time: 5 Minutes
Servings: 4

Nutrition:

Calories: 123
Carbs: 5g
Fat: 11g
Protein: 3g

Ingredients:

- 1 tbsp Extra virgin olive oil (1 tablespoon)
- 1 medium lemon
- ½ tsp Freshly grated nutmeg
- ½ tsp black pepper
- ½ tsp Kosher salt

Directions:

1. Warm the oven to 500°F. Put the asparagus on an aluminum

foil and drizzle with extra virgin olive oil, and toss until well coated.

2. Roast the asparagus in the oven for about five minutes; toss and continue roasting until browned. Sprinkle the roasted asparagus with nutmeg, salt, zest, and pepper.

Chicken Kale Wraps

Preparation Time: 10 Minutes
Cooking Time: 10 Minutes
Servings: 4
Nutrition:
Calories 106
Fat 5.1
Fiber 1.1
Carbs 6.3
Protein 9
Ingredients:

- 4 kale leaves
- 4 oz chicken fillet
- ½ apple
- 1 tablespoon butter
- ¼ teaspoon chili pepper
- ¾ teaspoon salt
- 1 tablespoon lemon juice
- ¾ teaspoon dried thyme

Directions:

1. Chop the chicken fillet into small cubes. Then mix up the chicken with chili pepper and salt.
2. Heat butter in the skillet. Add chicken cubes. Roast them for 4 minutes.
3. Meanwhile, chop the apple into small cubes and add to the chicken. Mix up well.
4. Sprinkle the ingredients with lemon juice and dried thyme. Cook them for 5 minutes over medium-high heat.
5. Fill the kale leaves with the hot chicken mixture and wrap.

Tomato Triangles

Preparation Time: 10 Minutes
Cooking Time: 0 Minutes
Servings: 6
Nutrition:
Calories 71
Fat 1.6
Fiber 2.1
Carbs 12.8
Protein 2.3
Ingredients:

- 6 corn tortillas
- 1 tablespoon cream cheese
- 1 tablespoon ricotta cheese
- ½ teaspoon minced garlic
- 1 tablespoon fresh dill, chopped
- 2 tomatoes, sliced

Directions:

1. Cut every tortilla into 2 triangles. Then mix up cream cheese, ricotta cheese, minced garlic, and dill.
2. Spread 6 triangles with cream cheese mixture.
3. Then place the sliced tomato on them and cover with remaining tortilla triangles. Serve.

Zaatar Fries

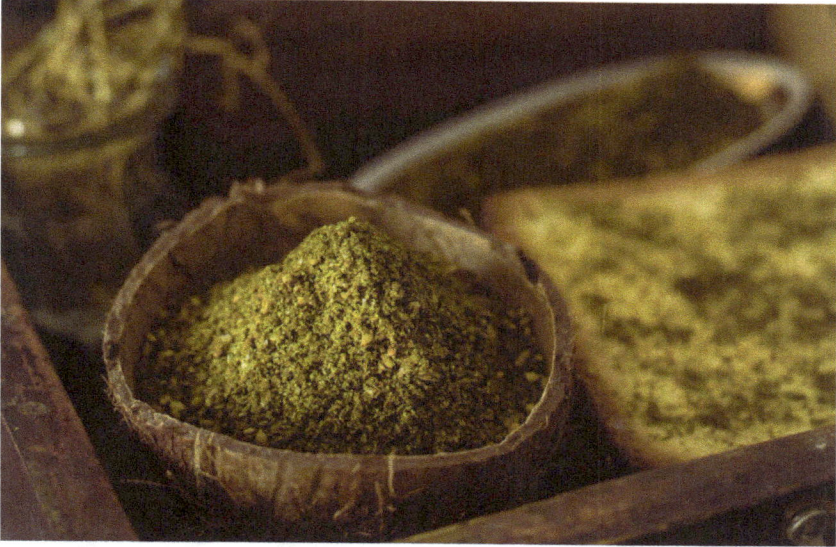

Preparation Time: 10 Minutes
Cooking Time: 35 Minutes
Servings: 5

Nutrition:
Calories 28
Fat 2.9
Fiber 0.2
Carbs 0.6
Protein 0.2
Ingredients:

- 1 teaspoon Zaatar spices
- 3 sweet potatoes
- 1 tablespoon dried dill
- 1 teaspoon salt
- 3 teaspoons sunflower oil
- ½ teaspoon paprika

Directions:

1. Pour water into the crockpot. Cut the sweet potatoes into fries.

2. Line the baking tray with parchment. Place the layer of the sweet potato in the tray.
3. Sprinkle the vegetables with dried dill, salt, and paprika. Then sprinkle sweet potatoes with Za'atar and mix up well with the help of the fingertips.
4. Sprinkle the sweet potato fries with sunflower oil—Preheat the oven to 375F.
5. Bake the sweet potato fries within 35 minutes. Stir the fries every 10 minutes.

Summertime Vegetable Chicken Wraps

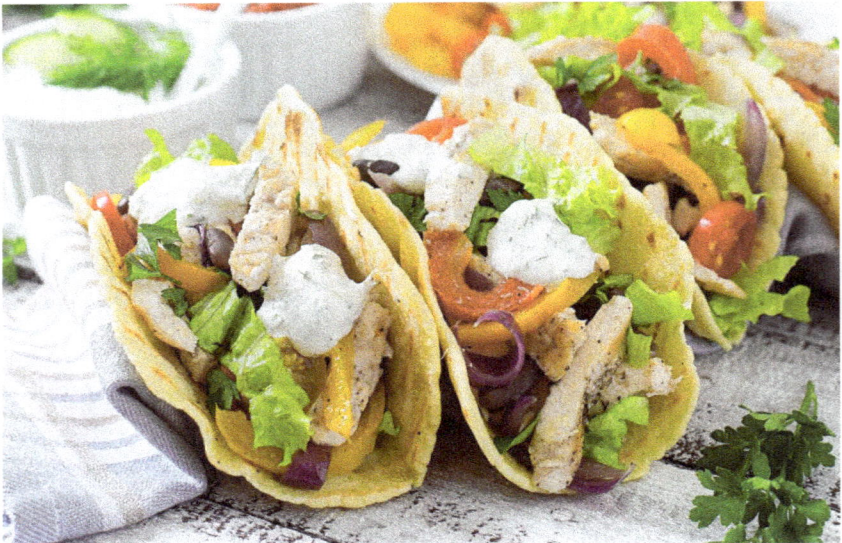

Preparation Time: 15 Minutes
Cooking Time: 0 Minutes
Servings: 4

Nutrition:
Calories: 278
Fat: 4g
Carbohydrates: 28g
Protein: 27g
Ingredients:

- 2 cups cooked chicken, chopped
- $\frac{1}{2}$ English cucumbers, diced
- $\frac{1}{2}$ red bell pepper, diced
- $\frac{1}{2}$ cup carrot, shredded
- 1 scallion, white and green parts, chopped
- $\frac{1}{4}$ cup plain Greek yogurt
- 1 tablespoon freshly squeezed lemon juice
- $\frac{1}{2}$ teaspoon fresh thyme, chopped
- Pinch of salt
- Pinch of ground black pepper
- 4 multigrain tortillas

Directions:

1. Take a medium bowl and mix in chicken, red bell pepper, cucumber, carrot, yogurt, scallion, lemon juice, thyme, sea salt and pepper.
2. Mix well.
3. Spoon one quarter of chicken mix into the middle of the tortilla and fold the opposite ends of the tortilla over the filling.
4. Roll the tortilla from the side to create a snug pocket.
5. Repeat with the remaining ingredients and serve.

Premium Roasted Baby Potatoes

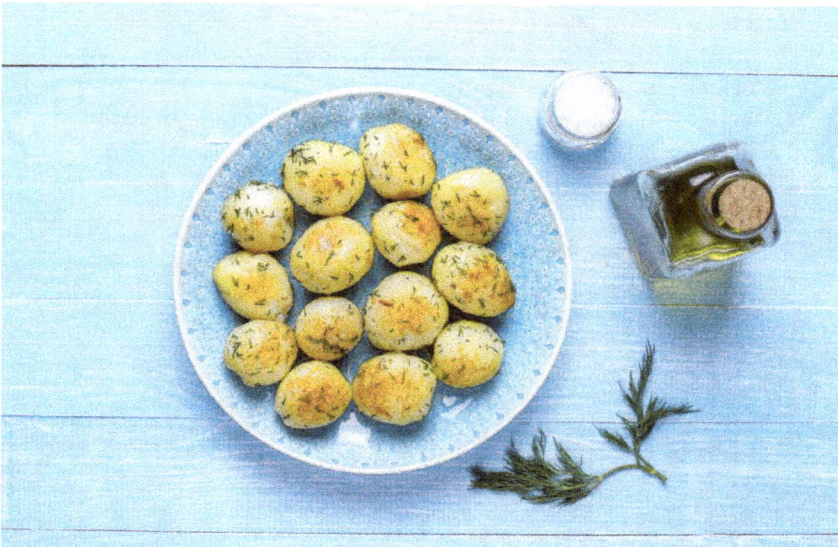

Preparation Time: 10 Minutes
Cooking Time: 35 Minutes
Servings: 4

Nutrition:
Calories: 225
Fat: 7g
Carbohydrates: 37g
Protein: 5g

Ingredients:

- 2 pounds new yellow potatoes, scrubbed and cut into wedges
- 2 tablespoons extra virgin olive oil
- 2 teaspoons fresh rosemary, chopped
- 1 teaspoon garlic powder
- 1 teaspoon sweet paprika
- ½ teaspoon sea salt
- ½ teaspoon freshly ground black pepper

Directions:

1. Pre-heat your oven to 400 degrees Fahrenheit.
2. Take a large bowl and add potatoes, olive oil, garlic, rosemary, paprika, sea salt and pepper.
3. Spread potatoes in single layer on baking sheet and bake for 35 minutes.
4. Serve and enjoy!

Tomato and Cherry Linguine

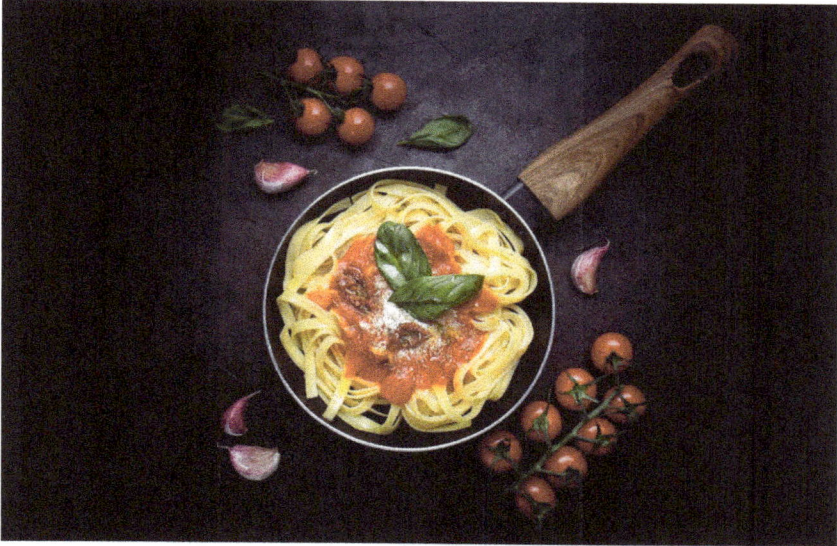

Preparation Time: 10 Minutes
Cooking Time: 15 Minutes
Servings: 4

Nutrition:
Calories: 397
Fat: 15g
Carbohydrates: 55g
Protein: 13g

Ingredients:

- 2 pounds cherry tomatoes
- 3 tablespoons extra virgin olive oil
- 2 tablespoons balsamic vinegar
- 2 teaspoons garlic, minced
- Pinch of fresh ground black pepper
- ¾ pound whole-wheat linguine pasta
- 1 tablespoon fresh oregano, chopped
- ¼ cup feta cheese, crumbled

Directions:

1. Pre-heat your oven to 350 degrees Fahrenheit.
2. Take a large bowl and add cherry tomatoes, 2 tablespoons olive oil, balsamic vinegar, garlic, pepper and toss.
3. Spread tomatoes evenly on baking sheet and roast for 15 minutes.
4. While the tomatoes are roasting, cook the pasta according to the package instructions and drain the paste into a large bowl.
5. Toss pasta with 1 tablespoon olive oil.
6. Add roasted tomatoes (with juice) and toss.
7. Serve with topping of oregano and feta cheese.

Mediterranean Zucchini Mushroom Pasta

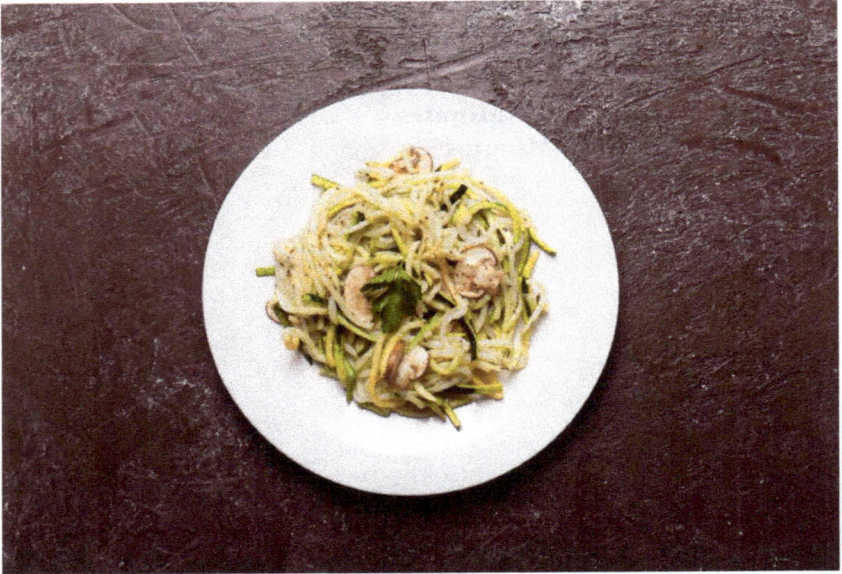

Preparation Time: 10 Minutes
Cooking Time: 10 Minutes
Servings: 4
Nutrition:
Calories: 361
Fat: 12g
Carbohydrates: 47g
Protein: 14g

. . .

Ingredients:

- ½ pound pasta
- 2 tablespoons olive oil
- 6 garlic cloves, crushed
- 1 teaspoon red chili
- 2 spring onions, sliced
- 3 teaspoons rosemary
- 1 large zucchini, cut in half
- 5 large portabella mushrooms
- 1 can tomatoes
- 4 tablespoons Parmesan cheese
- Fresh ground black pepper

Directions:

1. Cook the pasta.
2. Take a large-sized frying pan and place it over medium heat.
3. Add oil and allow the oil to heat up.
4. Add garlic, onion and chili and sauté for a few minutes until golden.
5. Add zucchini, rosemary and mushroom and sauté for a few minutes.
6. Increase the heat to medium-high and add tinned tomatoes to the sauce until thick.
7. Drain your boiled pasta and transfer to serving platter.
8. Pour the tomato mix on top and mix using tongs.
9. Garnish with Parmesan and freshly ground black pepper.

Lemon and Garlic Fettucine

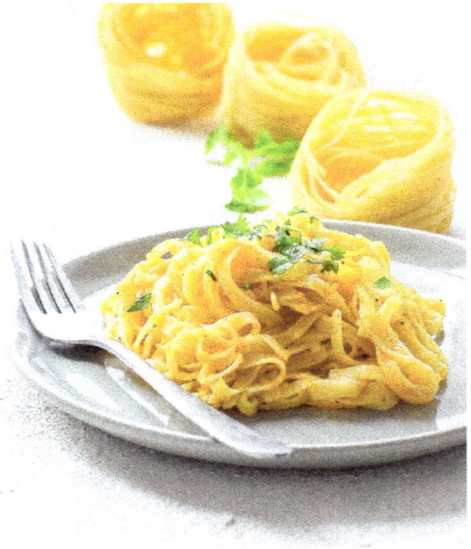

Preparation Time: 5 Minutes
Cooking Time: 15 Minutes
Servings: 5

Nutrition:
Calories: 480
Fat: 21g
Carbohydrates: 53g
Protein: 23g

Ingredients:

- 8 ounces of whole wheat fettuccine
- 4 tablespoons of extra virgin olive oil
- 4 cloves of minced garlic
- 1 cup of fresh breadcrumbs
- ¼ cup of lemon juice
- 1 teaspoon of freshly ground pepper
- ½ teaspoon of salt
- 2 cans of 4 ounce boneless and skinless sardines (dipped in tomato sauce)

- ½ cup of chopped up fresh parsley
- ¼ cup of finely shredded Parmesan cheese

Directions:

1. Take a large-sized pot and bring water to a boil.
2. Cook pasta for 10 minutes until Al Dente.
3. Take a small-sized skillet and place it over medium heat.
4. Add 2 tablespoons of oil and allow it to heat up.
5. Add garlic and cook for 20 seconds.
6. Transfer the garlic to a medium-sized bowl
7. Add breadcrumbs to the hot skillet and cook for 5-6 minutes until golden
8. Whisk in lemon juice, pepper and salt into the garlic bowl
9. Add pasta to the bowl (with garlic) and sardines, parsley and Parmesan
10. Stir well and sprinkle bread crumbs

Spinach and Feta Bread

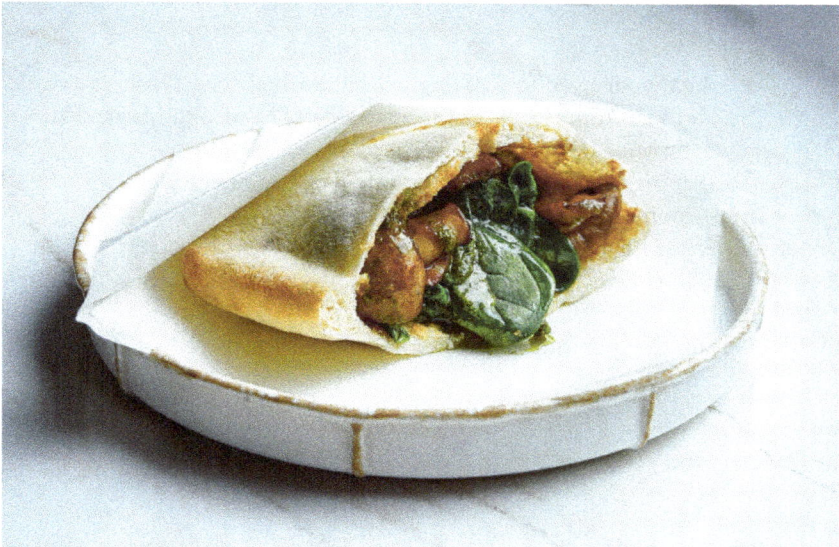

Preparation Time: 10 Minutes
Cooking Time: 12 Minutes
Servings: 6

. . .

Nutrition:

Calories: 350
Fat: 17g
Carbohydrates: 41g
Protein:11g

Ingredients:

- 6 ounces of sun-dried tomato pesto
- 6 pieces of 6-inch whole wheat pita bread
- 2 chopped up Roma plum tomatoes
- 1 bunch of rinsed and chopped spinach
- 4 sliced fresh mushrooms
- ½ cup of crumbled feta cheese
- 2 tablespoons of grated Parmesan cheese
- 3 tablespoons of olive oil
- Ground black pepper as needed

Directions:

1. Pre-heat your oven to 350 degrees Fahrenheit.
2. Spread your tomato pesto onto one side of your pita bread and place on your baking sheet (with the pesto side up).
3. Top up the pitas with spinach, tomatoes, feta cheese, mushrooms and Parmesan cheese.
4. Drizzle with some olive oil and season nicely with pepper.
5. Bake in your oven for around 12 minutes until the breads are crispy.
6. Cut up the pita into quarters and serve!

Roasted Broccoli with Parmesan

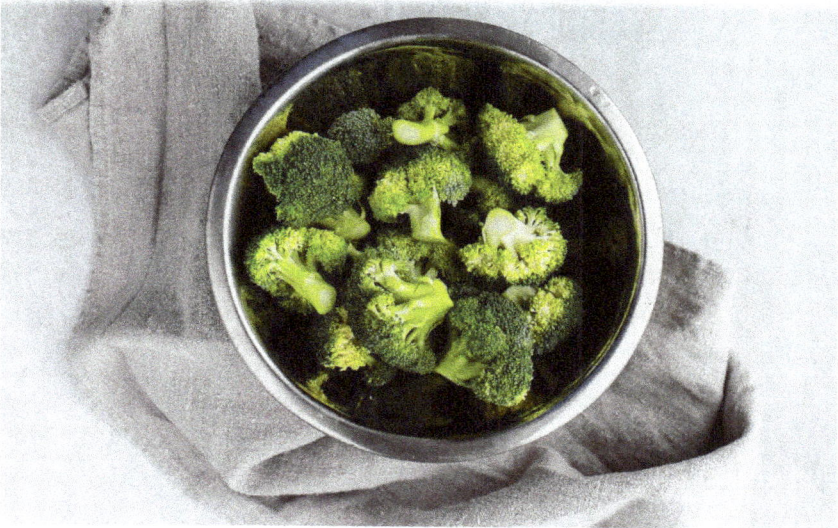

Preparation Time: 10 Minutes
Cooking Time: 10 Minutes
Servings: 4

Nutrition:
Calories: 154
Fat: 11g
Carbohydrates: 10g
Protein: 9g

Ingredients:

- 2 head broccolis, cut into florets
- 2 tablespoons extra-virgin olive oil
- 2 teaspoons garlic, minced
- Zest of 1 lemon
- Pinch of salt
- ½ cup Parmesan cheese, grated

Directions:

1. Pre-heat your oven to 400 degrees Fahrenheit.
2. Take a large bowl and add broccoli with 2 tablespoons olive oil, lemon zest, garlic, lemon juice and salt.
3. Spread mix on the baking sheet in single layer and sprinkle with Parmesan cheese.
4. Bake for 10 minutes until tender.
5. Transfer broccoli to serving the dish.

Quick Zucchini Bowl

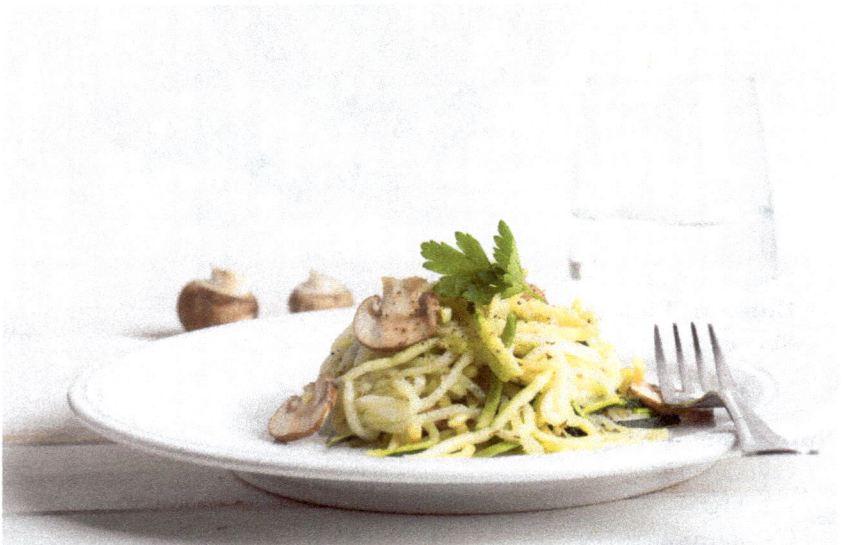

Preparation Time: 10 Minutes
Cooking Time: 10 Minutes
Servings: 4

Nutrition:
Calories: 361
Fat: 12g
Carbohydrates: 47g
Protein: 14g

Ingredients:

- ½ pound of pasta
- 2 tablespoons of olive oil
- 6 crushed garlic cloves
- 1 teaspoon of red chili
- 2 finely sliced spring onions
- 3 teaspoons of chopped rosemary
- 1 large zucchini cut up in half, lengthways and sliced
- 5 large portabella mushrooms
- 1 can of tomatoes
- 4 tablespoons of Parmesan cheese
- Fresh ground black pepper

Directions:

1. Cook the pasta.
2. Take a large-sized frying pan and place over medium heat.
3. Add oil and allow the oil to heat up.
4. Add garlic, onion and chili and sauté for a few minutes until golden.
5. Add zucchini, rosemary and mushroom and sauté for a few minutes.
6. Increase the heat to medium-high and add tinned tomatoes to the sauce until thick.
7. Drain your boiled pasta and transfer to a serving platter.
8. Pour the tomato mix on top and mix using tongs.
9. Garnish with Parmesan cheese and freshly ground black pepper.

Healthy Basil Platter

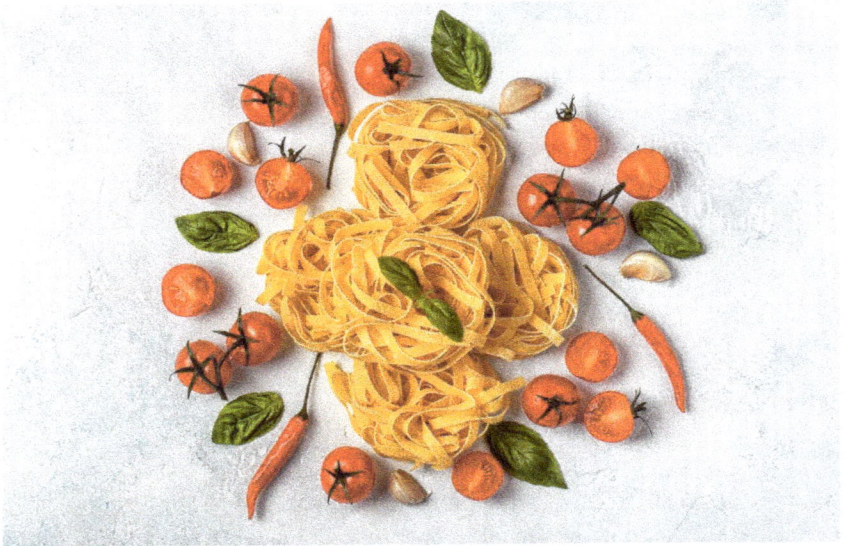

Preparation Time: 25 Minutes
Cooking Time: 15 Minutes
Servings: 4

Nutrition:
Calories: 452
Fat: 8g
Carbohydrates: 88g
Protein: 14g
Ingredients:

- 2 pieces of red pepper seeded and cut up into chunks
- 2 pieces of red onion cut up into wedges
- 2 mild red chilies, diced and seeded
- 3 coarsely chopped garlic cloves
- 1 teaspoon of golden caster sugar
- 2 tablespoons of olive oil (plus additional for serving)
- 2 pounds of small ripe tomatoes quartered up
- 12 ounces of dried pasta
- Just a handful of basil leaves
- 2 tablespoons of grated Parmesan

Directions:

1. Pre-heat the oven to 392 degrees Fahrenheit.
2. Take a large-sized roasting tin and scatter pepper, red onion, garlic and chilies.
3. Sprinkle sugar on top.
4. Drizzle olive oil then season with pepper and salt.
5. Roast the veggies in your oven for 15 minutes.
6. Take a large-sized pan and cook the pasta in boiling, salted water until Al Dente.
7. Drain them.
8. Remove the veggies from the oven and tip in the pasta into the veggies.
9. Toss well and tear basil leaves on top.
10. Sprinkle Parmesan and enjoy!

6

Lunch

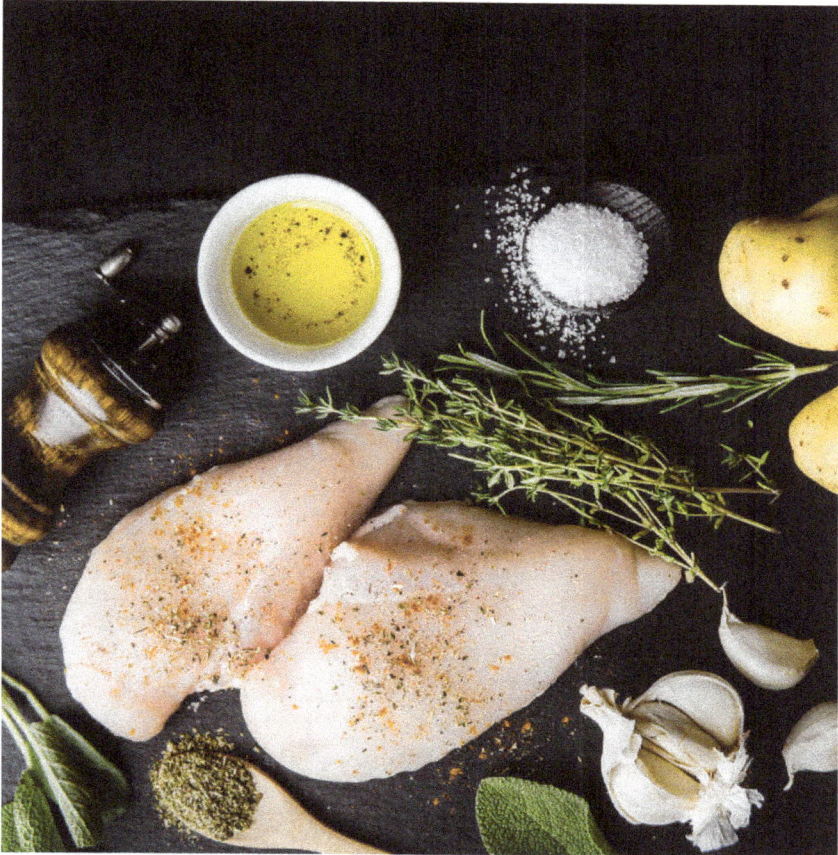

Turkey and Cranberry Sauce

Preparation Time: 10 Minutes
Cooking Time: 50 Minutes
Servings: 4
Nutrition:
Calories:382,
Fat:12.6,
Fiber:9.6,
Carbs:26.6,
Protein:17.6
Ingredients:

- 1 cup chicken stock
- 2 tablespoons avocado oil
- ½ cup cranberry sauce
- 1 big turkey breast, skinless, boneless and sliced
- 1 yellow onion, roughly chopped
- Salt and black pepper to the taste

Directions:

1. Heat up a pan with the avocado oil over medium-high heat, add the onion and sauté for 5 minutes.
2. Add the turkey and brown for 5 minutes more.
3. Add the rest of the ingredients, toss, introduce in the oven at 350 degrees F and cook for 40 minutes

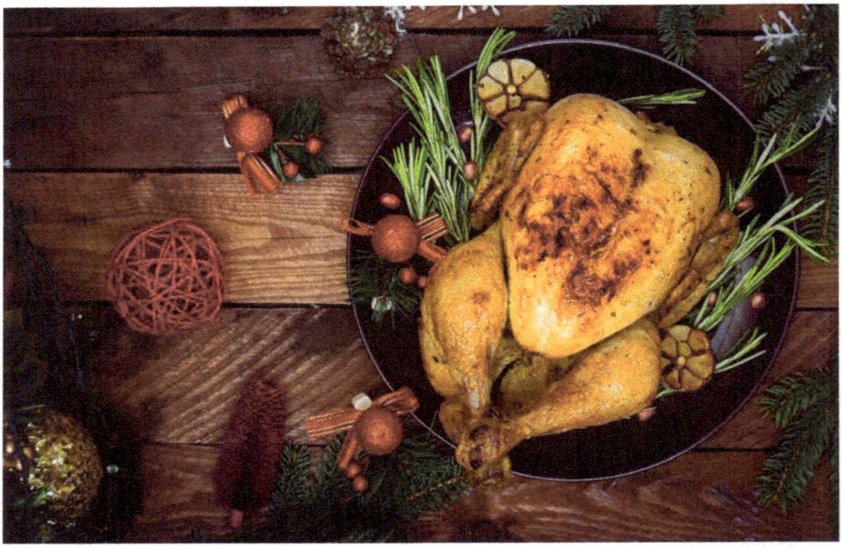

Sage Turkey Mix

Preparation Time: 10 Minutes
Cooking Time: 40 Minutes
Servings: 4
Nutrition:
Calories:382,

Fat:12.6,
Fiber:9.6,
Carbs:16.6,
Protein:33.2

Ingredients:

- 1 big turkey breast, skinless, boneless and roughly cubed
- Juice of 1 lemon
- 2 tablespoons avocado oil
- 1 red onion, chopped
- 2 tablespoons sage, chopped
- 1 garlic clove, minced
- 1 cup chicken stock

Directions:

1. Heat up a pan with the avocado oil over medium-high heat, add the turkey and brown for 3 minutes on each side.
2. Add the rest of the fixings, let it simmer and cook over medium heat for 35 minutes.
3. Divide the mix between plates and serve with a side dish.

Turkey and Asparagus Mix

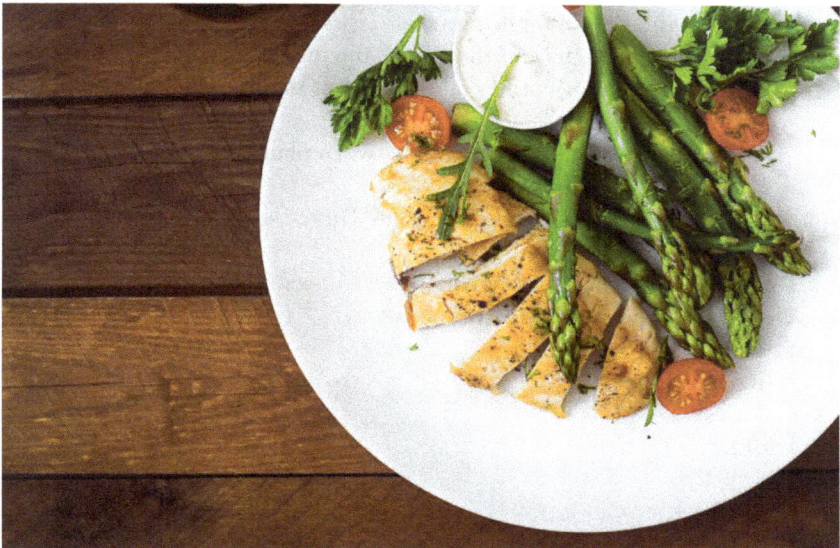

Preparation Time: 10 Minutes
Cooking Time: 30 Minutes
Servings: 4

Nutrition:
Calories:337,
Fat:21.2,
Fiber:10.2,
Carbs:21.4,
Protein:17.6
Ingredients:

- 1 bunch asparagus, trimmed and halved
- 1 big turkey breast, skinless, boneless and cut into strips
- 1 teaspoon basil, dried
- 2 tablespoons olive oil
- A pinch of salt and black pepper
- ½ cup tomato sauce
- 1 tablespoon chives, chopped

Directions:

1. Heat up a pan with the oil with medium heat, then put the turkey and brown for 4 minutes.
2. Add the asparagus and the rest of the ingredients except the chives, bring to a simmer and cook over medium heat for 25 minutes.
3. Add the chives, divide the mix between plates and serve.

Herbed Almond Turkey

Preparation Time: 10 Minutes
Cooking Time: 40 Minutes
Servings: 4
Nutrition:
Calories:297,
Fat:11.2,
Fiber:9.2,
Carbs:19.4,
Protein:23.6

Ingredients:

- 1 big turkey breast, skinless, boneless and cubed
- 1 tablespoon olive oil
- ½ cup chicken stock
- 1 tablespoon basil, chopped
- 1 tablespoon rosemary, chopped
- 1 tablespoon oregano, chopped
- 1 tablespoon parsley, chopped
- 3 garlic cloves, minced
- ½ cup almonds, toasted and chopped
- 3 cups tomatoes, chopped

Directions:

1. Warmth up a pan through the oil over medium-high heat, add the turkey and the garlic and brown for 5 minutes.
2. Add the stock in addition the rest of the fixings, bring to a simmer over medium heat and cook for 35 minutes.
3. Divide the mix between plates and serve.

Thyme Chicken

Preparation Time: 10 Minutes
Cooking Time: 50 Minutes
Servings: 4
Nutrition:
Calories:281,
Fat:9.2,
Fiber:10.9,
Carbs:21.6,
Protein:13.6
Ingredients:

- 1 tablespoon olive oil
- 4 garlic cloves, minced
- A pinch of salt and black pepper
- 2 teaspoons thyme, dried
- 12 small red potatoes, halved
- 2 pounds chicken breast, skinless, boneless and cubed

- 1 cup red onion, sliced
- ¾ cup chicken stock
- 2 tablespoons basil, chopped

Directions:

1. In a baking dish greased with the oil, add the potatoes, chicken and the rest of the ingredients, toss a bit, introduce in the oven and bake at 400 degrees F for 50 minutes.

Turkey, Artichokes and Asparagus

Preparation Time: 10 Minutes
Cooking Time: 30 Minutes
Servings: 4
Nutrition:
Calories:291,
Fat:16,
Fiber:10.3,
Carbs:22.8,
Protein:34.5
Ingredients:

- 2 turkey breasts, boneless, skinless and halved
- 3 tablespoons olive oil
- 1 and ½ pounds asparagus, trimmed and halved
- 1 cup chicken stock
- A pinch of salt and black pepper
- 1 cup canned artichoke hearts, drained
- ¼ cup kalamata olives, pitted and sliced
- 1 shallot, chopped
- 3 garlic cloves, minced
- 3 tablespoons dill, chopped

Directions:

1. Warmth up a pan through the oil over medium-high heat, add the turkey and the garlic and brown for 4 minutes on each side.
2. Add the asparagus, the stock and the rest of the ingredients

except the dill, bring to a simmer and cook over medium heat for 20 minutes. Add the dill and serve.

Lemony Turkey and Pine Nuts

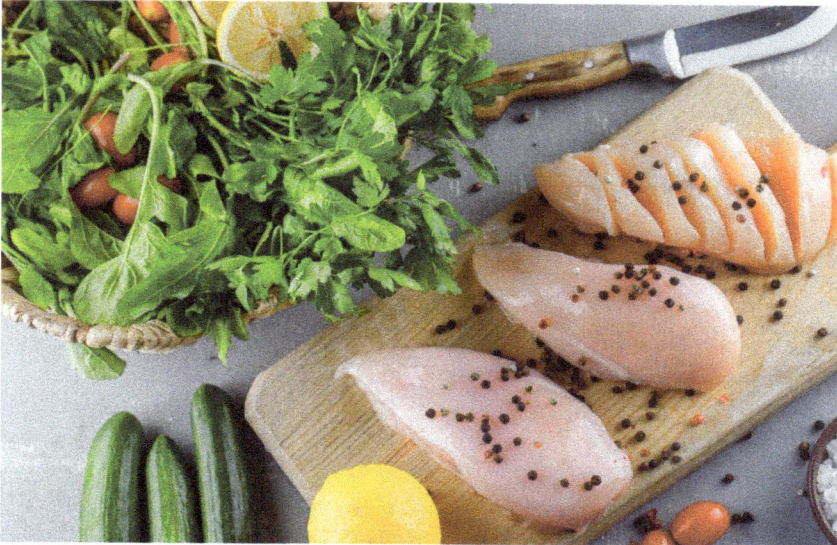

Preparation Time: 10 Minutes
Cooking Time: 30 Minutes
Servings: 4

Nutrition:
Calories:293,
Fat:12.4,
Fiber:9.3,
Carbs:17.8,
Protein:24.5
Ingredients:

- 2 turkey breasts, boneless, skinless and halved
- A pinch of salt and black pepper
- 2 tablespoons avocado oil
- Juice of 2 lemons
- 1 tablespoon rosemary, chopped

- 3 garlic cloves, minced
- ¼ cup pine nuts, chopped
- 1 cup chicken stock

Directions:

1. Warmth up a pan through the oil over medium-high heat, add the garlic and the turkey and brown for 4 minutes on each side.
2. Add the rest of the fixings, let it simmer and cook over medium heat for 20 minutes.
3. Divide the mix between plates and serve with a side salad.

Yogurt Chicken and Red Onion Mix

Preparation Time: 10 Minutes
Cooking Time: 30 Minutes
Servings: 4
Nutrition:
Calories:278,
Fat:15,
Fiber:9.2,
Carbs:15.1,
Protein:23.3
Ingredients:

- 2 pounds chicken breast, skinless, boneless and sliced
- 3 tablespoons olive oil
- ¼ cup Greek yogurt
- 2 garlic cloves, minced
- ½ teaspoon onion powder
- A pinch of salt and black pepper
- 4 red onions, sliced

Directions:

1. In a roasting pan, combine the chicken with the oil, the yogurt and the other ingredients, introduce in the oven at 375 degrees F and bake for 30 minutes.
2. Divide chicken mix between plates and serve hot.

Chicken and Mint Sauce

Preparation Time: 10 Minutes
Cooking Time: 30 Minutes
Servings: 4
Nutrition:
Calories:278,
Fat;12,
Fiber:11.2,
Carbs:18.1,
Protein:13.3
Ingredients:

- 2 and ½ tablespoons olive oil
- 2 pounds chicken breasts, skinless, boneless and halved
- 3 tablespoons garlic, minced
- 2 tablespoons lemon juice
- 1 tablespoon red wine vinegar
- 1/3 cup Greek yogurt
- 2 tablespoons mint, chopped
- A pinch of salt and black pepper

Directions:

1. Blend the garlic plus lemon juice and the other ingredients except the oil and the chicken and pulse well.
2. Warmth up a pan through the oil over medium-high heat, add the chicken and brown for 3 minutes on each side.
3. Add the mint sauce, introduce in the oven and bake everything at 370 degrees F for 25 minutes.

Chicken and Sausage Mix

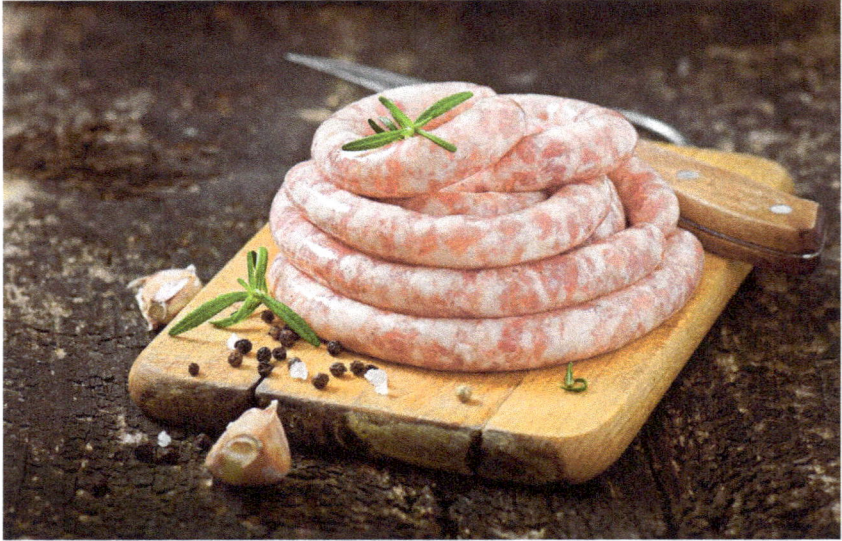

Preparation Time: 10 Minutes
Cooking Time: 50 Minutes
Servings: 4
Nutrition:
Calories:293,
Fat:13.1,
Fiber:8.1,
Carbs:16.6,
Protein:26.1

Ingredients:

- 2 zucchinis, cubed
- 1-pound Italian sausage, cubed
- 2 tablespoons olive oil
- 1 red bell pepper, chopped
- 1 red onion, sliced
- 2 tablespoons garlic, minced
- 2 chicken breasts, boneless, skinless and halved
- Salt and black pepper to the taste
- ½ cup chicken stock
- 1 tablespoon balsamic vinegar

Directions:

1. Heat up a pan with half of the oil over medium-high heat, add the sausages, brown for 3 minutes on each side and transfer to a bowl.
2. Heat up the pan again with the rest of the oil over medium-high heat, add the chicken and brown for 4 minutes on each side.
3. Return the sausage, add the rest of the ingredients as well, bring to a simmer, introduce in the oven and bake at 400 degrees F for 30 minutes.
4. Divide everything between plates and serve.

Oregano Turkey and Peppers

Preparation Time: 10 Minutes
Cooking Time: 1 Hour
Servings: 4
Nutrition:
Calories:229,
Fat:8.9,
Fiber:8.2,
Carbs:17.8,
Protein:33.6
Ingredients:

- 2 red bell peppers, cut into strips
- 2 green bell peppers, cut into strips
- 1 red onion, chopped
- 4 garlic cloves, minced
- ½ cup black olives, pitted and sliced
- 2 cups chicken stock
- 1 big turkey breast, skinless, boneless and cut into strips
- 1 tablespoon oregano, chopped
- ½ cup cilantro, chopped

Directions:

1. In a baking pan, combine the peppers with the turkey and the rest of the ingredients, toss, introduce in the oven at 400 degrees F and roast for 1 hour.

2. Divide everything between plates and serve.

Chicken and Mustard Sauce

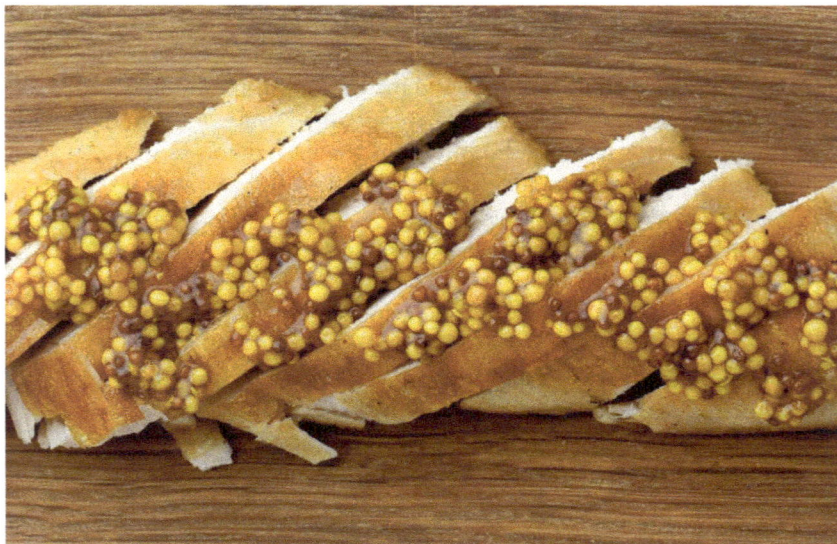

Preparation Time: 10 Minutes
Cooking Time: 26 Minutes
Servings: 4

Nutrition:
Calories:247,
Fat:15.1,
Fiber:9.1,
Carbs:16.6,
Protein:26.1
Ingredients:

- 1/3 cup mustard
- Salt and black pepper to the taste
- 1 red onion, chopped
- 1 tablespoon olive oil
- 1 and ½ cups chicken stock
- 4 chicken breasts, skinless, boneless, and halved

- ¼ teaspoon oregano, dried

Directions:

1. Heat up a pan with the stock over medium heat, add the mustard, onion, salt, pepper and the oregano, whisk, bring to a simmer and cook for 8 minutes.
2. Warmth up a pan through the oil over medium-high heat, add the chicken and brown for 3 minutes on each side.
3. Add chicken into the pan with the sauce, toss, simmer everything for 12 minutes more, divide between plates and serve.

Coriander and Coconut Chicken

Preparation Time: 10 Minutes
Cooking Time: 30 Minutes
Servings: 4
Nutrition:
Calories:297,
Fat:14.4,
Fiber:9.6,
Carbs:22,
Protein:25
Ingredients:

- 2 pounds chicken thighs, skinless, boneless and cubed
- 2 tablespoons olive oil
- Salt and black pepper to the taste
- 3 tablespoons coconut flesh, shredded
- 1 and ½ teaspoons orange extract
- 1 tablespoon ginger, grated
- ¼ cup orange juice
- 2 tablespoons coriander, chopped
- 1 cup chicken stock
- ¼ teaspoon red pepper flakes

Directions:

1. Warmth up a pan through the oil over medium-high heat, add the chicken and brown for 4 minutes on each side.

2. Add salt, pepper and the rest of the ingredients, bring to a simmer and cook over medium heat for 20 minutes.
3. Divide the mix between plates and serve hot.

Saffron Chicken Thighs and Green Beans

Preparation Time: 10 Minutes
Cooking Time: 25 Minutes
Servings: 4
Nutrition:
Calories:274,
Fat:12.3,
Fiber:5.3,
Carbs:20.4,
Protein:14.3
Ingredients:

- 2 pounds chicken thighs, boneless and skinless
- 2 teaspoons saffron powder
- 1-pound green beans, trimmed and halved
- ½ cup Greek yogurt
- Salt and black pepper to the taste
- 1 tablespoon lime juice
- 1 tablespoon dill, chopped

Directions:

1. In a roasting pan, combine the chicken with the saffron, green beans and the rest of the ingredients, toss a bit, introduce in the oven and bake at 400 degrees F for 25 minutes.

Chicken and Olives Salsa

Preparation Time: 10 Minutes
Cooking Time: 25 Minutes
Servings: 4
Nutrition:
Calories:289,
Fat:12.4,
Fiber:9.1,
Carbs:23.8,

Protein:14.3
Ingredients:

- 2 tablespoon avocado oil
- 4 chicken breast halves, skinless and boneless
- Salt and black pepper to the taste
- 1 tablespoon sweet paprika
- 1 red onion, chopped
- 1 tablespoon balsamic vinegar
- 2 tablespoons parsley, chopped
- 1 avocado, peeled, pitted and cubed
- 2 tablespoons black olives, pitted and chopped

Directions:

1. Heat up your grill over medium-high heat, add the chicken brushed with half of the oil and seasoned with paprika, salt and pepper, cook for 7 minutes on each side and divide between plates.
2. Meanwhile, in a bowl, mix the onion with the rest of the ingredients and the remaining oil, toss, add on top of the chicken and serve.

Carrots and Tomatoes Chicken

Preparation Time: 10 Minutes
Cooking Time: 1 Hour 10 Minutes
Servings: 4
Nutrition:
Calories:309,
Fat:12.4,
Fiber:11.1,
Carbs:23.8,
Protein:15.3
Ingredients:

- 2 pounds chicken breasts, skinless, boneless and halved
- Salt and black pepper to the taste
- 3 garlic cloves, minced
- 3 tablespoons avocado oil

- 2 shallots, chopped
- 4 carrots, sliced
- 3 tomatoes, chopped
- ¼ cup chicken stock
- 1 tablespoon Italian seasoning
- 1 tablespoon parsley, chopped

Directions:

1. Warmth up a pan through the oil over medium-high heat, add the chicken, garlic, salt and pepper and brown for 3 minutes on each side.
2. Add the rest of the fixings excluding the parsley, bring to a simmer and cook over medium-low heat for 40 minutes.

Smoked and Hot Turkey Mix

Preparation Time: 10 Minutes
Cooking Time: 40 Minutes
Servings: 4
Nutrition:
Calories:310,
Fat:18.4,
Fiber:10.4,
Carbs:22.3,
Protein:33.4
Ingredients:

- 1 red onion, sliced
- 1 big turkey breast, skinless, boneless and roughly cubed
- 1 tablespoon smoked paprika
- 2 chili peppers, chopped
- Salt and black pepper to the taste
- 2 tablespoons olive oil
- ½ cup chicken stock
- 1 tablespoon parsley, chopped
- 1 tablespoon cilantro, chopped

Directions:

1. Grease a roasting pan through the oil, add the turkey, onion,

paprika and the rest of the ingredients, toss, introduce in the oven and bake at 425 degrees F for 40 minutes.

2. Divide the mix between plates and serve right away.

Spicy Cumin Chicken

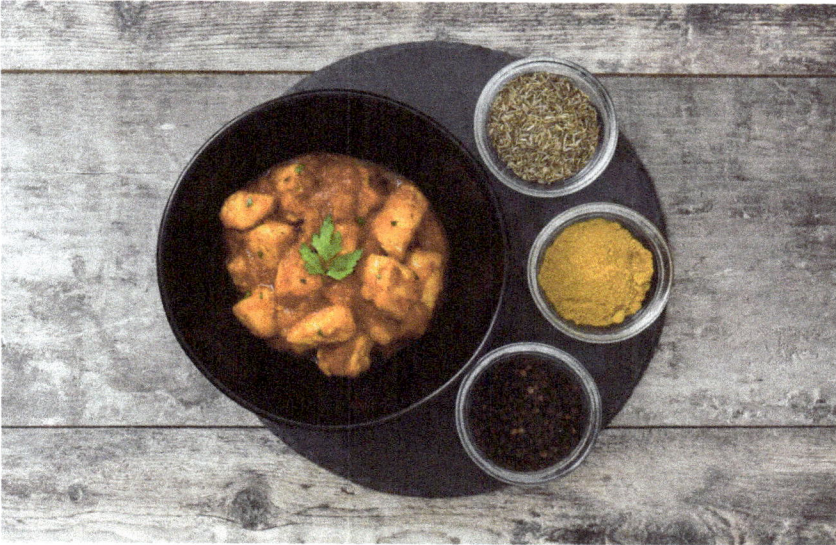

Preparation Time: 10 Minutes
Cooking Time: 25 Minutes
Servings: 4

Nutrition:
Calories:230,
Fat:18.4,
Fiber:9.4,
Carbs:15.3,
Protein:13.4
Ingredients:

- 2 teaspoons chili powder
- 2 and ½ tablespoons olive oil
- Salt and black pepper to the taste
- 1 and ½ teaspoons garlic powder

- 1 tablespoon smoked paprika
- ½ cup chicken stock
- 1-pound chicken breasts, skinless, boneless and halved
- 2 teaspoons sherry vinegar
- 2 teaspoons hot sauce
- 2 teaspoons cumin, ground
- ½ cup black olives, pitted and sliced

Directions:

1. Warm up a pan with the oil over medium-high heat, add the chicken and brown for 3 minutes on each side.
2. Add the chili powder, salt, pepper, garlic powder and paprika, toss and cook for 4 minutes more.
3. Add the rest of the ingredients, toss, bring to a simmer and cook over medium heat for 15 minutes more.

Chicken with Artichokes and Beans

Preparation Time: 10 Minutes
Cooking Time: 40 Minutes
Servings: 4
Nutrition:
Calories:291,
Fat:14.9,
Fiber:10.5,
Carbs:23.8,
Protein:24.2
Ingredients:

- 2 tablespoons olive oil
- 2 chicken breasts, skinless, boneless and halved
- Zest of 1 lemon, grated
- 3 garlic cloves, crushed
- Juice of 1 lemon
- Salt and black pepper to the taste
- 1 tablespoon thyme, chopped
- 6 ounces canned artichokes hearts, drained
- 1 cup canned fava beans, drained and rinsed
- 1 cup chicken stock
- A pinch of cayenne pepper

Directions:

1. Warmth up a pan with the oil on medium-high heat, add chicken and brown for 5 minutes.
2. Add lemon juice, lemon zest, salt, pepper and the rest of the ingredients, bring to a simmer and cook over medium heat for 35 minutes.
3. Divide the mix between plates and serve right away.

Chicken and Olives Tapenade

Preparation Time: 10 Minutes
Cooking Time: 25 Minutes
Servings: 4
Nutrition:
Calories:291,
Fat:12.9,
Fiber:8.5,
Carbs:15.8,
Protein:34.2
Ingredients:

- 2 chicken breasts, boneless, skinless and halved
- 1 cup black olives, pitted
- ½ cup olive oil
- Salt and black pepper to the taste
- ½ cup mixed parsley, chopped
- ½ cup rosemary, chopped
- Salt and black pepper to the taste
- 4 garlic cloves, minced
- Juice of ½ lime

Directions:

1. In a blender, combine the olives with half of the oil and the rest of the ingredients except the chicken and pulse well.
2. Heat up a pan with the rest of the oil over medium-high heat, add the chicken and brown for 4 minutes on each side.
3. Add the olives mix, and cook for 20 minutes more tossing often.

Lunch

Mexican Tacos

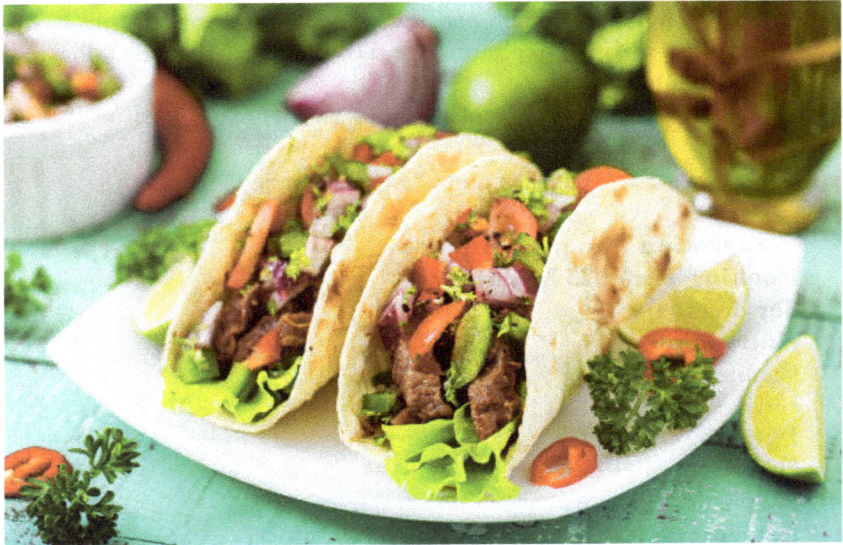

If you are looking for a spicy and comforting lunch option for both you and your family or friends, then these Mexican tacos are just what you need. The recipe makes 7 servings, which means you can store them for up to 3 days in the refrigerator for the week, or enjoy them among a group of people.

Time: 30 minutes

Serving Size: 7 (2 tacos each)

Prep Time: 20 minutes

Cook Time: 10 minutes

Nutritional Info:

Calories: 340

Carbs: 32 g

Fat: 15 g

Protein: 19 g

Sodium: 494 mg

Potassium: 422 mg

Phosphorus: 276 mg

Ingredients:

- 14 6-inch flour tortillas
- 1 oz ground beef

- 2 cups of lettuce
- ½ cup of tomato sauce (low-sodium)
- 5 tbsp of onions
- 5 tbsp of sour cream
- 5 tbsp of mozzarella cheese
- 1 tbsp of olive oil
- Mexican seasoning: 3 tsp chili powder, 2 tsp paprika, 2 tsp ground cumin, 1 tsp onion powder, ½ tsp of garlic powder, and ⅛ tsp of black pepper.

Directions:

1. Prepare the Mexican seasoning recipe by combining the paprika, ground cumin, onion powder, garlic powder, chili powder, and black pepper.
2. Chop the lettuce and onion into small pieces.
3. On a medium non-stick pan, add 1 tbsp of olive oil and cook the ground beef for a few minutes until it is golden brown. Once done, add the seasoning mixture and the tomato sauce.
4. Place the tortillas in the microwave oven and heat for 20 seconds until they are slightly warm.
5. Assemble the soft tacos by dividing the ground beef mixture evenly between all 14 of the tortillas.
6. Add 1 tsp of mozzarella cheese, 1 tsp of onion, 1 tsp of sour cream, and lettuce to each taco. Serve the tacos warm.

Food-prep tip: Store the tacos in airtight containers and place them in the refrigerator for up to 3 days.

Strawberry Sandwich

Who doesn't like a good sandwich — and who knew you could make the perfect one with strawberries? This is a very low-protein and low-calorie lunch option that can be enjoyed on the go. It is quick to make and easy to pack, and low in potassium and phosphorus to support any kidney condition, including dialysis.

Time: 5 minutes
Serving Size: 1
Prep Time: 5 minutes
Cook Time: 0 minutes
Nutritional Info:
Calories: 123
Carbs: 18.5 g
Fat: 3.7 g
Protein: 4 g

Sodium: 200.8 mg

Potassium: 75.2 mg

Phosphorus: 44.2 mg

Ingredients:

- 2 slices of whole-wheat sandwich bread
- 2 medium strawberries (sliced)
- 1 tbsp of cream cheese (reduced-fat)
- ¼ tsp of honey
- ⅛ tsp of orange zest (freshly grated)

Directions:

1. Combine the cream cheese, orange zest, and honey in a small bowl.
2. Plate the two slices of bread and spread them with the cheese mixture.
3. Add the strawberry slices on top of one bread slice, and close it with the other to make a sandwich.

Food-prep tip: Prep your strawberry sandwich for the next day's lunch the night before. Seal it in a Ziploc bag or an airtight plastic container in the refrigerator.

Crunch Chicken Wraps

For a high-quality protein option and a source of healthy fats, this burrito is filling and meets all your health requirements, no matter the kidney condition you may be struggling with. It also is low in carbs and calories.

Time: 10 minutes

Serving Size: 4

Prep Time: 5 minutes

Cook Time: 5 minutes

Nutritional Info:

Calories: 315

Carbs: 15 g

Fat: 21.4 g

Protein: 17.2 g

Sodium: 107.9 mg

Potassium: 480 mg

Phosphorus: 385 mg

Ingredients:

- 4 large tortillas
- 1 avocado
- 2 cups of cooked chicken breasts (shredded)

- ½ cup of mozzarella cheese
- 2 tbsp of cilantro (chopped)
- 1 tbsp of olive oil

Directions:

1. Prep a batch of chicken breasts cooked for 40 minutes at 180°F, then shred and store in the refrigerator in an airtight container.
2. Add the shredded chicken, diced avocado, cilantro, and mozzarella cheese to a medium bowl.
3. Place the tortillas flat on 4 separate plates, and add a ¼ of the chicken filling mixture.
4. Hand-roll each burrito.
5. Warm 1 tbsp of olive oil in a large non-stick pan over medium heat and add the burritos. Flip the burritos, cooking them for 1 minute on each side or until they are golden brown. Serve them warm.

Food-prep tip: Store the burritos for the week in an airtight container to enjoy as a lunch option on the go or at home. To save time, prep the chicken over the weekend to last you for meals for the week ahead.

Chicken and Broccoli Stromboli

This pizza-dough bread dish is like a hug on a cold winter's day. It's packed with nutrients and a high-quality source of protein that is also low in fat.

Time: 35 minutes
Serving Size: 4
Prep Time: 15 minutes
Cook Time: 20 minutes
Nutritional Info:
Calories: 522
Carbs: 52 g
Fat: 5 g
Protein: 38 g
Sodium: 607 mg
Potassium: 546 mg
Phosphorus: 400 mg
Ingredients:

- 1 oz of pizza dough (store-bought)
- 2 cups of cooked chicken breast (diced)
- 2 cups of broccoli florets (fresh and blanched)
- 1 cup of cheddar cheese (shredded)
- 2 tbsp of olive oil

- 1 tbsp oregano (chopped)
- 1 tbsp of garlic (chopped)
- 1 tbsp of flour
- 1 tsp of red pepper flakes (crushed)

Directions:

1. Preheat the oven to 400°F.
2. Mix the chicken, broccoli, garlic, pepper flakes, and oregano in a bowl, and set aside.
3. Dust a clean, flat tabletop surface with flour. Roll out the dough until it has reached a rectangular shape of 11" x 14".
4. Add the chicken mixture 2 inches from the dough's edge on the longer side. Roll and pinch the dough's ends, seaming it until it is tightly sealed. This can be done with a fork or the back of a coffee mug.
5. Brush the top of the dough with olive oil. Follow this by making 3 small slits at the top part of the dough.
6. Bake the dish on a lightly oiled baking tray for 10 to 12 minutes, or until it is golden brown.
7. Remove the stromboli from the oven and let it sit for 5 minutes before serving it hot.

Food-prep tip: Store the remaining stromboli in an airtight container, or cover the baking dish to seal with tin foil. It will keep in the refrigerator for up to 3 days.

Shrimp Quesadilla

This shrimp dish is filled with quality ingredients and makes a fit source of protein for anyone with a kidney condition or diabetes. It is low in carbs, low in protein, and will keep you full and satisfied until dinner.

Time: 20 minutes
Serving Size: 2
Prep Time: 10 minutes
Cook Time: 10 minutes
Nutritional Info:
Calories: 318
Carbs: 26 g
Fat: 15 g
Protein: 20 g
Sodium: 398 mg
Potassium: 276 mg
Phosphorus: 243 mg
Ingredients:

- 5 oz of shrimp (raw)
- 2 flour tortillas
- 2 tbsp of cilantro
- 2 tbsp of cheddar cheese (shredded)
- 2 tbsp of sour cream
- 1 tbsp lemon juice
- 4 tsp of salsa
- ¼ tsp of cumin
- ⅛ tsp of cayenne pepper

Directions:

1. Shell and devein the shrimp, followed by rinsing and cutting it into bite-sized pieces.
2. Chop the cilantro finely and combine it with lemon juice, cayenne pepper, and cumin in a Ziploc bag to make a marinade. Place the shrimp pieces in the bag, and allow it to sit for 5 minutes.
3. Heat a medium non-stick skillet over medium heat and add the shrimp with the remaining marinade to the skillet. Stir-fry the contents for 2 minutes, or until the shrimp turns orange. Once done, remove the skillet from the heat. Spoon the shrimp out of the marinade into a separate bowl.
4. Add sour cream to your marinade in a skillet, and then stir to mix it.
5. Heat the tortillas in the microwave for 30 seconds to a minute.
6. Spread 2 tsp of salsa onto each of the tortillas before topping it with ½ of the seasoned shrimp.
7. Sprinkle each tortilla with 1 tbsp of cheese, and spoon the sour cream mixture onto the shrimp.
8. Fold the tortilla in half to close and place it on a new skillet for a few seconds. Turn the tortilla over when it becomes slightly golden brown. Repeat this step with the other tortilla, as well.
9. Cut the tortillas into 4 pieces each, and garnish with a little cilantro and a lemon wedge to serve.

Food-prep tip: Store the tortillas in airtight sealed glass containers in the refrigerator for up to 2 days.

BBQ Chicken Pita

Who doesn't love a BBQ chicken combo for a meal? Even with CKD, dialysis, general poor kidney function, or diabetes, you can enjoy this pizza alternative, which is low in calories, fat, and offers a high-quality source of protein.

Time: 15 minutes
Serving Size: 2
Prep Time: 3 minutes
Cook Time: 12 minutes
Nutritional Info:
Calories: 320
Carbs: 37 g
Fat: 9 g
Protein: 23 g
Sodium: 523 mg
Potassium: 255 mg
Phosphorus: 221 mg
Ingredients:
- 2 6" pita bread
- 4 oz of chicken (cooked, cubed)
- ¼ cup of purple onion (sliced)
- 3 tbsp of barbecue sauce (low-sodium)
- 2 tbsp of feta cheese
- ⅛ tsp of garlic powder

Directions:

1. Preheat the oven to 350°F.
2. Prepare a baking sheet by spraying it with a layer of non-stick cooking spray.
3. Place 2 pitas on the sheet, followed by 1 ½ tbsp of barbecue sauce on each of the pitas.
4. Top with onion slices and cubed chicken, then sprinkle feta and garlic powder over the pitas.
5. Bake the pitas in the oven for 12 minutes before removing them and allowing them to cool down slightly before serving.

Food-prep tip: Slice the pitas into smaller pieces, and store them in a sealed, airtight glass container in the refrigerator for up to 3 days.

Mediterranean Bean Salad

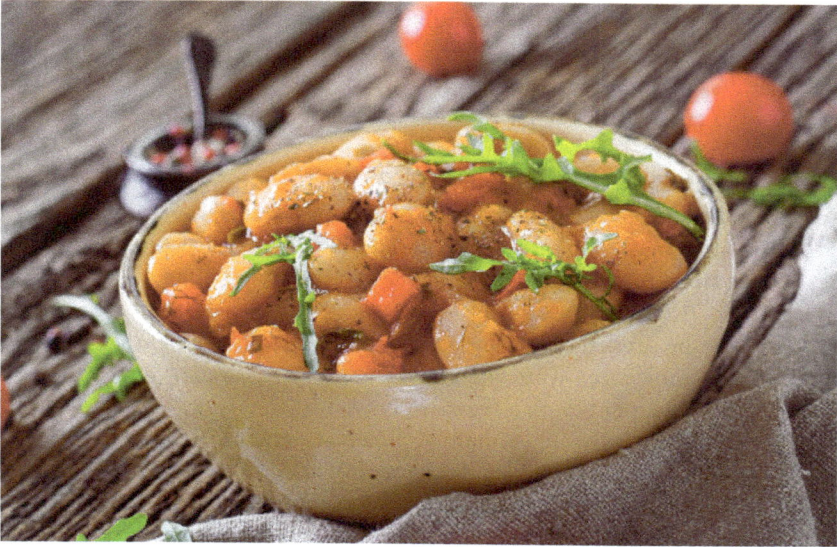

As a light, and quick-to-make lunch, this bean salad is a step outside of the box from your traditional bowl of greens. It has a combination of delicious flavors and will leave you feeling fresh and satisfied. The salad can be served on its own as a main dish, or as a side to a good source of protein like chicken or fish. The meal is low in protein and calories.

Time: 20 minutes

Serving Size: 8

Prep Time: 20 minutes

Cook Time: 0 minutes

Nutritional Info:

Calories: 308

Carbs: 35 g

Fat: 15 g

Protein: 13 g

Sodium: 924 mg

Potassium: 500 mg

Phosphorus: 323 mg

Ingredients:

- 1 can of cannellini beans (19 oz, drained and rinsed)
- 1 can of kidney beans (19 oz, drained and rinsed)
- 1 can of chickpeas (15 oz, drained and rinsed)
- 1/2 of an English cucumber (quartered and sliced)
- 1 red bell pepper (diced)
- 1 cup of rosa tomatoes (sliced)

- ¾ cup of feta cheese (crumbled)
- ½ cup of olives (sliced)
- ½ cup of red onion (diced)
- ½ cup of fresh parsley (chopped)
- 2 tbsp of fresh basil (chopped)
- Dressing: ⅓ cup of olive oil, 2 cloves of garlic, 3 tbsp of lemon juice (freshly squeezed), 3 tbsp of red wine vinegar, 2 tsp of dijon mustard, ½ tsp of oregano, ½ tsp of sea salt, and a pinch of black pepper.

Directions:

1. Mix the dressing ingredients, including the olive oil, garlic, lemon juice, red wine vinegar, dijon mustard, oregano, sea salt, and black pepper, in a medium bowl.
2. Combine the beans, tomato, bell pepper, cucumber, olives, red onion, basil, and parsley in a large bowl.
3. Once done, pour the salad dressing over the bean salad and toss all the ingredients until everything is well coated. Add the feta once done.
4. Cover the salad and allow it to rest to get the best flavor. Alternatively, it can be served right away.

Food-prep tip: Store the salad in an airtight glass container in the refrigerator for up to 3 days.

Sloppy Joe Turkey Burger

This burger is guilt-free, offers a good source of protein, and is low in potassium and phosphorus to provide you with a kidney-friendly meal option that is packed with nutrients and tastes more like a treat than a healthy meal! So, if you're feeling any cravings coming on, this is just the traditional burger alternative for you.

Time: 25 minutes
Serving Size: 6
Prep Time: 10 minutes
Cook Time: 15 minutes
Nutritional Info:
Calories: 290
Carbs: 28 g
Fat: 9 g
Protein: 24 g
Sodium: 288 mg
Potassium: 513 mg
Phosphorus: 237 mg
Ingredients:

- 6 hamburger buns
- 1 cup of tomato sauce (low-sodium)
- ½ cup of red onion (diced)
- ½ cup of yellow bell pepper (diced)
- 1 ½ oz of ground turkey (only 7% fat)
- 2 tbsp of brown sugar
- 1 tbsp of chicken seasoning
- 1 tbsp of Worcestershire sauce

Directions:

1. In a large non-stick pan over medium heat, cook the ground turkey until it is cooked through. Do not drain the pan once cooked.
2. Add the chicken seasoning, tomato sauce, Worcestershire sauce, and brown sugar to a small bowl, and mix the ingredients until well combined.
3. Add the seasonings to the mixture, followed by the diced vegetables.
4. Reduce the heat for the turkey dish to simmer, and continue to cook it for 10 minutes.
5. Divide the turkey mixture into 6 equal portions.
6. Spread 1 tbsp of cream cheese on both sides of the hamburger bun and add a portion of turkey mixture on top of each.

Food-prep tip: Store the leftover hamburgers in a sealed, airtight container in the refrigerator for up to 3 days.

Herb-Roasted Chicken With Vegetables

For a low-protein and weight-loss diet-friendly option, this roasted dish is the go-to lunch for you.

Time: 55 minutes
Serving Size: 4
Prep Time: 10 minutes
Cook Time: 45 minutes
Nutritional Info:
Calories: 215
Carbs: 8 g
Fat: 7 g
Protein: 30 g
Sodium: 107 mg
Potassium: 580 mg
Phosphorus: 250 mg
Ingredients:

- 8 garlic cloves (minced)
- 4 chicken breasts
- 2 medium zucchini (sliced ¼-inch thick)
- 1 medium carrot (sliced ¼-inch thick)
- ½ of yellow bell pepper (sliced ¼-inch thick)
- ½ of red onion (cut into ½-inch wedges)
- 1 tbsp of olive oil
- 1 tbsp dried cilantro
- ¼ tsp of pepper

Directions:

1. Preheat the oven to 375°F.
2. Add the zucchini, bell pepper, carrot, onion, and garlic in a roasting pan and drizzle the olive oil on top.
3. Season the vegetable mixture with black pepper and mix it with a spatula to coat. Roast the vegetables for about 10 minutes.
4. In the meantime, remove the skin from the chicken, and rub the meat with black pepper and cilantro. Place the skin back on and season with added pepper and rosemary as per your preference.
5. Remove the roasting dish from the oven and place the chicken breasts onto the vegetables. Place it back in the oven to continue roasting for 35 minutes.
6. Once done, remove the dish from the oven to cool down a little before serving it.

Food-prep tip: Place the leftovers in an airtight container and keep it refrigerated for lunch for the entire week. Store it for up to 4 days.

Seafood Noodle Salad

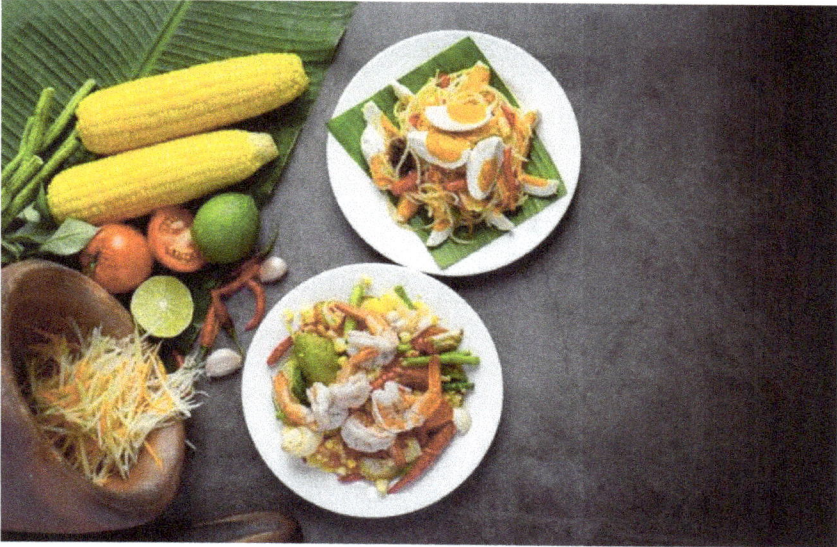

For a quick and easy Asian-inspired meal, this noodle salad recipe is packed with high-quality protein, but in a low quantity.

Time: 20 minutes
Serving Size: 10
Prep Time: 20 minutes
Cook Time: 0 minutes
Nutritional Info:
Calories: 254
Carbs: 27 g
Fat: 11 g
Protein: 13 g
Sodium: 433 mg
Potassium: 325 mg
Phosphorus: 229 mg
Ingredients:
- 1 oz of dry spaghetti (cooked and chilled, not rinsed)
- 4 cups of cocktail shrimp (peeled, deveined, tailless, and cooked)
- 2 cups of fresh broccoli florets
- 2 cups of button mushrooms (chopped)
- 1 ½ cups of water
- 1 cup of scallions (sliced)
- 1 cup of fresh carrots (shredded)
- ½ cup of red wine vinegar
- 2 tbsp of sesame oil

- 2 tsp of green tabasco
- 2 tbsp of fresh garlic (chopped)
- 1 tbsp of ginger (chopped)
- 1 tbsp of soy sauce
- ¼ cup of fresh lime juice
- zest of 1 lime
- 4 tsp of chicken base
- 4 tsp of balsamic vinegar
- 2 tsp of dark molasses
- ¼ tsp of ginger
- ¼ tsp of black pepper
- ¼ tsp of garlic powder

Directions:

1. Mix the spaghetti, cocktail shrimp, scallions, broccoli, carrots, and mushrooms in a large bowl. Set aside for later.
2. Blend the red wine vinegar, sesame oil, tabasco, garlic, ginger, soy sauce, lime juice and zest, chicken base, balsamic vinegar, dark molasses, ginger, black pepper, and garlic in a blender for 1 minute. The texture of the final product should be smooth.
3. Pour the dressing over the pasta mixture, and toss all of the ingredients together until it is well coated to serve.

Food-prep tip: Store the vegetable and shrimp noodle salad in a glass airtight container for up to 4 days. Prep it on Sunday night for lunch meals for the next week.

Lunch

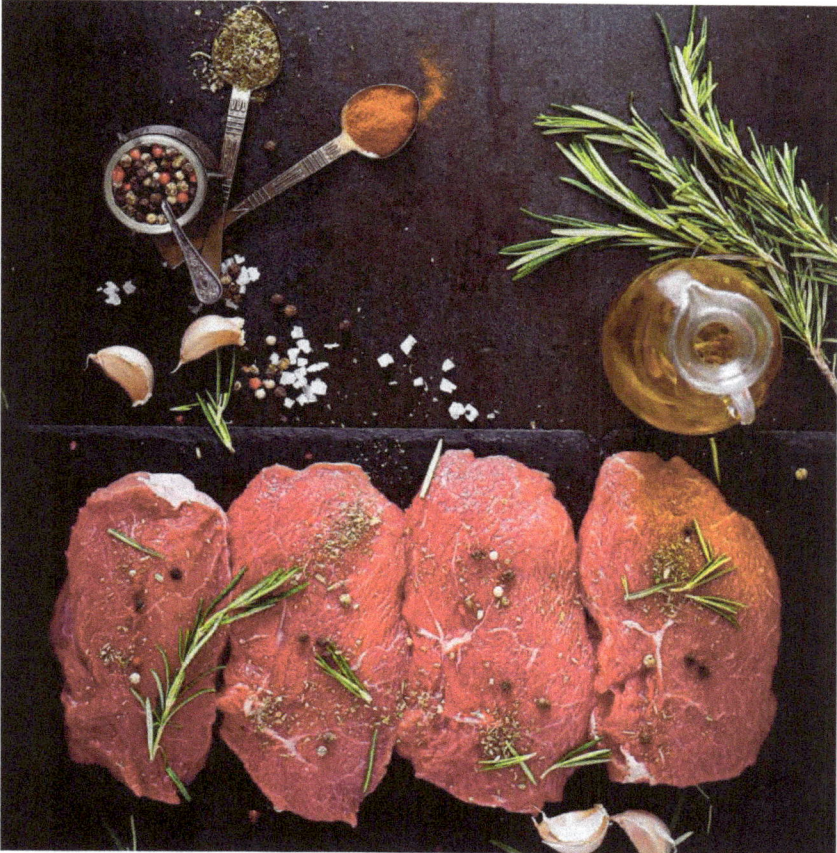

Tender Lamb Chops

Preparation Time: 10 Minutes
Cooking Time: 3 Hours
Servings: 4
Nutrition:
Calories 210
Fat 4.1 g
Carbohydrates 7.3 g
Protein 20.4 g
Ingredients:

- 8 lamb chops

- ½ teaspoon dried thyme
- 1 onion, sliced
- 1 teaspoon dried oregano
- 2 garlic cloves, minced
- 4 baby carrots
- Pepper and salt
- 2 potatoes, cubed
- 8 small tomatoes, halved

Directions:

1. Add the onion, carrots, tomatoes and potatoes into a pot.
2. Combine together thyme, oregano, pepper, and salt. Rub over lamb chops.
3. Place lamb chops in the pot and top with garlic.
4. Pour ¼ cup water around the lamb chops.
5. Cover and cook on low flame for around 3 hours.
6. Uncover the pot and roast at high flame for 10 minutes.
7. Serve and enjoy.

Beef Stroganoff

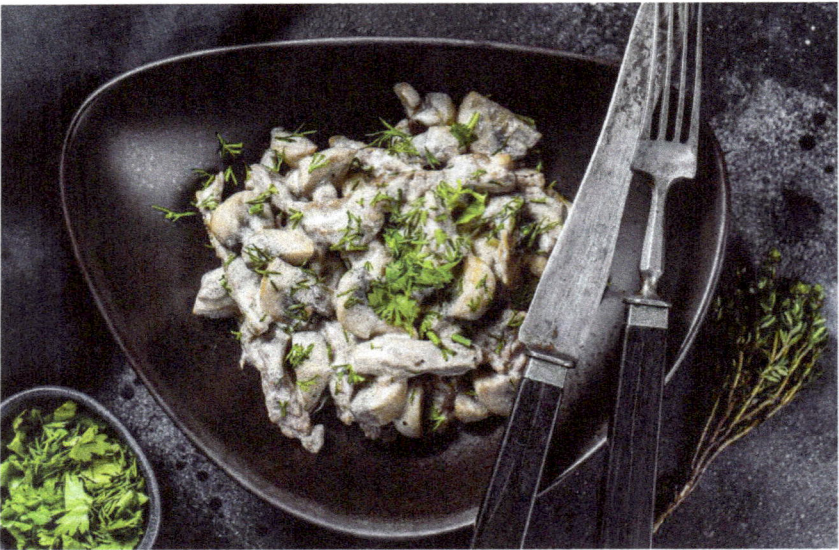

Preparation Time: 10 Minutes
Cooking Time: 4 Hours

Servings: 2

Nutrition:
Calories 470
Fat 25 g
Carbohydrates 8.6 g
Protein 49 g

Ingredients:

- 1/2 lb. beef stew meat
- 10 oz mushroom soup, homemade
- 1 medium onion, chopped
- 1/2 cup sour cream
- 1 oz mushrooms, sliced
- Pepper and salt

Directions:

1. Add all fixings excluding sour cream into a pot and mix well.
2. Cover and cook on low flame for 4 hours.
3. Add sour cream and stir well.
4. Serve and enjoy.

Lamb & Couscous Salad

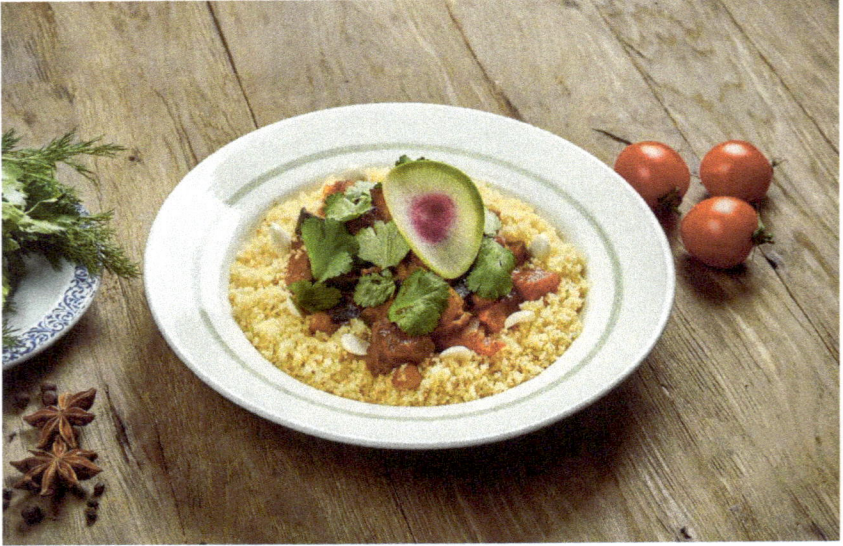

Preparation Time: 7 Minutes
Cooking Time: 25 Minutes
Servings: 2

Nutrition:
Calories: 232,
Fat: 7.9g,
Protein: 5.6g,
Carbohydrates: 31.2g

Ingredients:

- 1/2 Cup Water
- 1/2 Tablespoon Garlic, Minced
- 1 1/4 lb. Lamb Loin Chops, Trimmed
- 1/4 Cup Couscous, Whole Wheat
- Pinch Sea Salt
- 1/2 Tablespoon Parsley, Fresh & Chopped Fine
- 1 Tomato, Chopped
- 1 Teaspoon Olive Oil
- 1 Small Cucumber, Chopped

- 1 1/2 Tablespoons Lemon Juice, Fresh
- 1/4 Cup Feta, Crumbled
- 1 Tablespoon Dill, Fresh & Chopped Fine

Directions:

1. Get out a saucepan and bring the water to a boil.
2. Get out a bowl and mix your garlic, salt and parsley. Press this mixture into the side of each lamb chop, and then heat your oil using medium-high heat in a skillet.
3. Add the lamb, cooking for six minutes per side. Place it to the side, and cover to help keep the lamb chops warm.
4. Stir the couscous into the water once it's started to boil, returning it to a boil before reducing it to low so that it simmers. Cover, and then cook for about two minutes more. Take away from heat, then allow it to stand uncovered for five minutes. Fluff using a fork, and then add in your tomatoes, lemon juice, feta and dill. Stir well. Serve on the side of your lamb chops.

Smoky Pork & Cabbage

Preparation Time: 10 Minutes
Cooking Time: 3 Hours
Servings: 6
Nutrition:
Calories 484
Fat 21.5 g
Carbohydrates 4 g
Protein 36 g
Ingredients:

- 3lb pork
- 1/2 cabbage head, chopped
- 1 cup water
- 1/3 cup liquid smoke
- 1 tablespoon kosher salt

Directions:

1. Rub the pork with kosher salt and place into a pot.

2. Pour liquid smoke over the pork. Add water.
3. Cover then cook on low flame for 2 hours.
4. Remove pork from the pot and add cabbage in the bottom.
5. Place pork on top of the cabbage.
6. Cover again and cook for 1 hour more.
7. Slice the pork and serve.

Lemon Beef

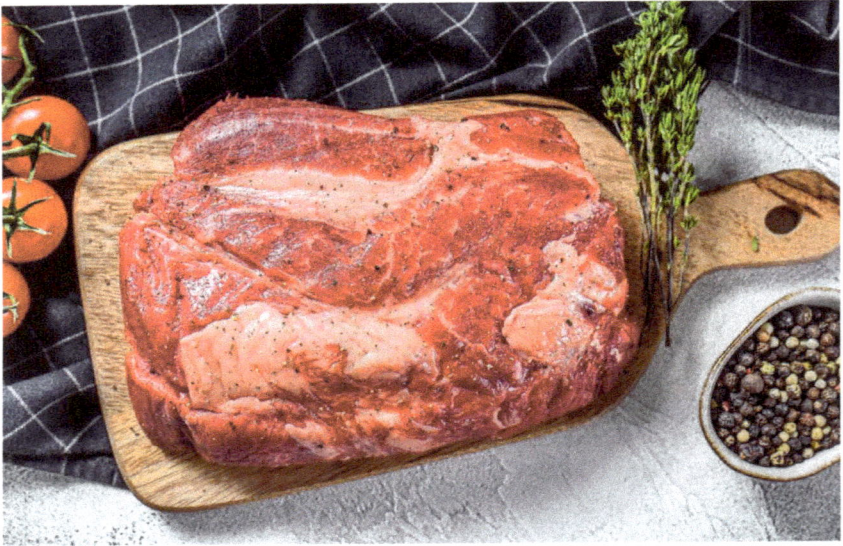

Preparation Time: 10 Minutes
Cooking Time: 3 Hours
Servings: 4
Nutrition:
Calories 355
Fat 16.8 g
Carbohydrates 14 g
Protein 35.5 g

Ingredients:

- 1 lb. beef chuck roast
- 1 fresh lime juice
- 1 garlic clove, crushed
- 1 teaspoon chili powder
- 2 cups lemon-lime soda
- 1/2 teaspoon salt

Directions:

1. Place beef chuck roast into a pot.
2. Season roast with garlic, chili powder, and salt.
3. Pour lemon-lime soda over the roast.
4. Cover the pot then cook on low flame for 3 hours. Shred the meat using fork.
5. Add lime juice over shredded roast and serve.

Herb Pork Roast

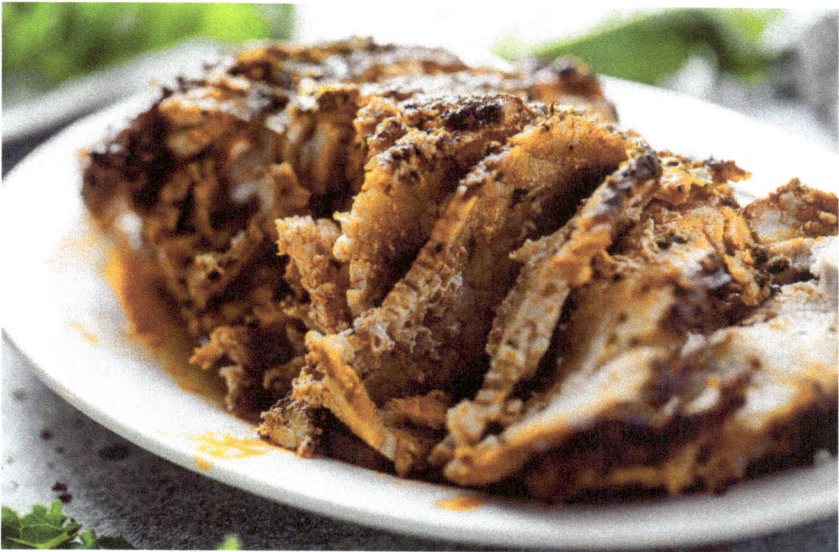

Preparation Time: 10 Minutes
Cooking Time: 2 Hours
Servings: 8

Nutrition:

Calories 327
Fat 8 g
Carbohydrates 0.5 g
Protein 59 g

Ingredients:

- 5 lbs. pork roast, boneless or bone-in
- 1 tablespoon dry herb mix
- 4 garlic cloves, cut into slivers
- 1 tablespoon salt

Directions:

1. By means of a sharp knife make small slices all over meat then insert garlic slivers into the cuts.
2. In a small bowl, mix together Italian herb mix and salt and rub all over pork roast.
3. Place the pork roast into a pot.
4. Cover then cook on low flame for 2 hours.
5. Uncover the pot and roast at high flame for 10 minutes.
6. Take away the meat from the pot and slice it.
7. Serve and enjoy.

Seasoned Pork Chops

Preparation Time: 10 Minutes
Cooking Time: 4 Hours
Servings: 4
Nutrition:
Calories 386
Fat 32.9 g
Carbohydrates 3 g
Protein 20 g
Ingredients:

- 4 pork chops
- 2 garlic cloves, minced
- 1 cup chicken broth

- 1 tablespoon poultry seasoning
- 1/4 cup olive oil
- Pepper and salt

Directions:

1. In a bowl, whisk together olive oil, poultry seasoning, garlic, broth, pepper, and salt.
2. Pour olive oil mixture into the slow cooker then place pork chops in the pot.
3. Cover and cook on low flame for about 3 hours.
4. Uncover the pot and roast at high flame for 10 minutes.
5. Dress the pork in the cooking sauce and serve along with vegetables.

Greek Beef Roast

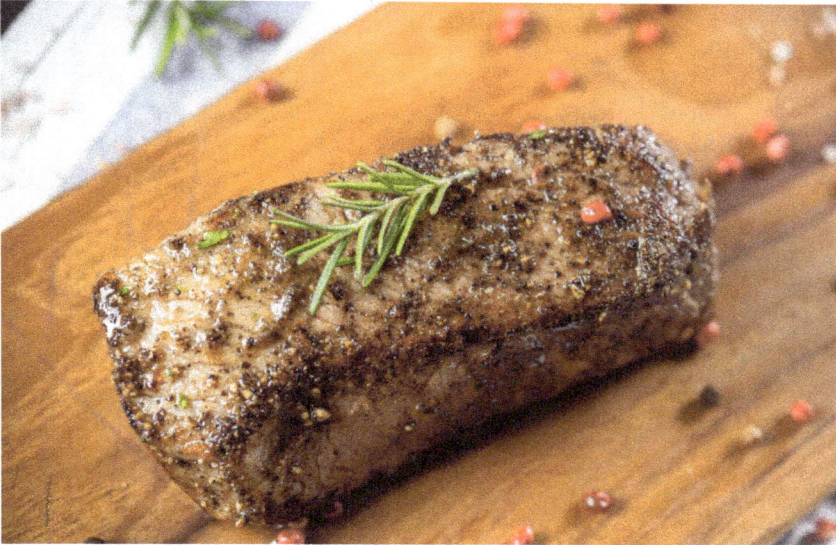

Preparation Time: 10 Minutes
Cooking Time: 2 Hours
Servings: 6
Nutrition:
Calories 231

Fat 6 g
Carbohydrates 4 g
Protein 35 g

Ingredients:

- 2 lbs. lean top round beef roast
- 1 tablespoon Italian seasoning
- 6 garlic cloves, minced
- 1 onion, sliced
- 2 cups beef broth
- $\frac{1}{2}$ cup red wine
- 1 teaspoon red pepper flakes
- Pepper
- Salt

Directions:

1. Season meat with pepper and salt and place into a pot.
2. Pour remaining ingredients over meat.
3. Cover then cook on low flame for 2 hours.
4. Slice the meat, dress with cooking sauce and serve.

Tomato Pork Chops

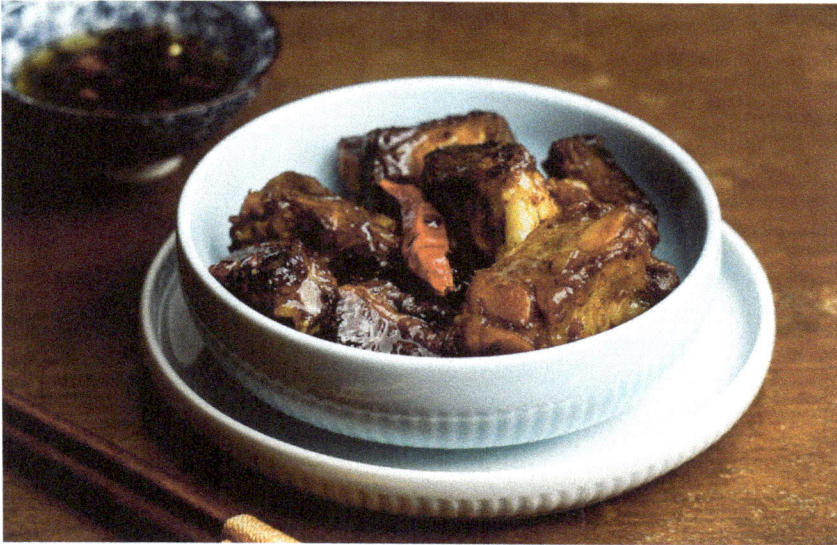

Preparation Time: 10 Minutes
Cooking Time: 1 Hour 10 Minutes
Servings: 4
Nutrition:
Calories 325
Fat 23.4 g
Carbohydrates 10 g
Protein 20 g

Ingredients:

- 4 pork chops, bone-in
- 1 tablespoon garlic, minced
- ½ small onion, chopped
- 6 oz can tomato paste
- 1 bell pepper, chopped
- ¼ teaspoon red pepper flakes
- 1 teaspoon Worcestershire sauce
- 1 tablespoon dried Italian seasoning
- 14.5 oz can tomato, diced

- 2 teaspoon olive oil
- ¼ teaspoon pepper
- 1 teaspoon kosher salt

Directions:

1. Warmth oil in a pan over medium-high heat.
2. Season pork chops with pepper and salt.
3. Sear pork chops in pan until brown from both the sides.
4. Transfer the pork chops into a pot.
5. Add the remaining ingredients to the pot.
6. Cover and cook on low flame for 1 hour.
7. Remove the lid and roast for about 10 minutes.

Pork Roast

Preparation Time: 10 Minutes
Cooking Time: 1 Hour 35 Minutes
Servings: 6
Nutrition:
Calories 502
Fat 23.8 g
Carbohydrates 3 g
Protein 65 g
Ingredients:

- 3 lbs. pork roast, boneless
- 1 cup water
- 1 onion, chopped
- 3 garlic cloves, chopped
- 1 tablespoon black pepper
- 1 rosemary sprig
- 2 fresh oregano sprigs
- 2 fresh thyme sprigs
- 1 tablespoon olive oil
- 1 tablespoon kosher salt

Directions:

1. Preheat the oven to 350 F.
2. Season pork roast with pepper and salt.

3. Heat olive oil in a stockpot and sear pork roast on each side, about 4 minutes.
4. Add onion and garlic. Pour in the water, oregano, and thyme and bring to boil for a minute.
5. Cover pot and roast in the preheated oven for 1 1/2 hours.

Greek Pork Chops

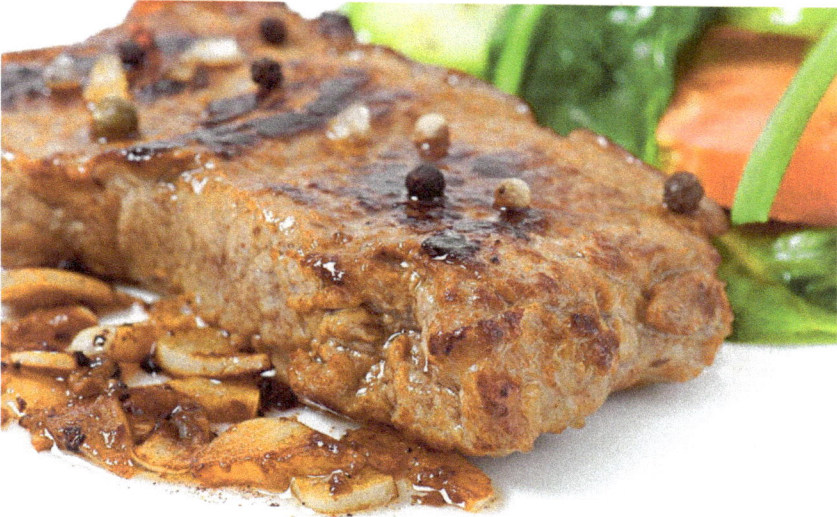

Preparation Time: 10 Minutes
Cooking Time: 15 Minutes
Servings: 4
Nutrition:
Calories 324
Fat 26.5 g
Carbohydrates 2.5 g
Sugar 1.3 g
Protein 18 g
Cholesterol 69 mg

Ingredients:

- 8 pork chops, boneless
- 4 teaspoon dried oregano
- 2 tablespoon Worcestershire sauce
- 3 tablespoon fresh lemon juice
- ¼ cup olive oil
- 1 teaspoon ground mustard
- 2 teaspoon garlic powder
- 2 teaspoon onion powder
- Pepper
- Salt

Directions:

1. Whisk together oil, garlic powder, onion powder, oregano, Worcestershire sauce, lemon juice, mustard, pepper, and salt.
2. Place pork chops in a baking dish then pour marinade over pork chops and coat well. Place in refrigerator overnight.
3. Preheat the grill.
4. Place pork chops on hot grill and cook for 7-8 minutes on each side.

Pork Cacciatore

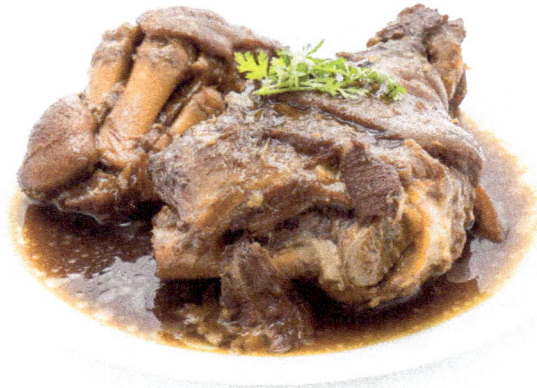

Preparation Time: 10 Minutes
Cooking Time: 2 Hours
Servings: 4
Nutrition:
Calories 440
Fat 33 g
Carbohydrates 6 g
Protein 28 g

Ingredients:

- 1 ½ lbs. pork chops
- 1 teaspoon dried oregano
- 1 cup beef broth
- 3 tablespoon tomato paste
- 14 oz can tomato, diced
- 2 cups mushrooms, sliced
- 1 small onion, diced
- 1 garlic clove, minced
- 2 tablespoon olive oil
- ¼ teaspoon pepper
- ½ teaspoon salt

Directions:

1. Warmth oil in a pan over medium-high heat.
2. Add pork chops in pan and cook until brown on both the sides.
3. Transfer pork chops into a pot.
4. Pour remaining ingredients over the pork chops.
5. Cover then cook on low flame for 2 hours.

Easy Beef Kofta

Preparation Time: 10 Minutes
Cooking Time: 10 Minutes
Servings: 6
Nutrition:
Calories 223
Fat 7.3 g

Carbohydrates 2.5 g

Protein 35 g

Ingredients:

- 2 lbs. ground beef
- 4 garlic cloves, minced
- 1 onion, minced
- 2 teaspoon cumin
- 1 cup fresh parsley, chopped
- ¼ teaspoon pepper
- 1 teaspoon salt
- 1 tablespoon oil

Directions:

1. With a knife, chop the beef very well.
2. Add all the fixings excluding oil into the mixing bowl and mix until combined.
3. Roll meat mixture into mini-kabab shapes.
4. Add the oil to a pan then warm up at high flame.
5. Roast the meat in the hot pan for 4-6 minutes on each side or until cooked.
6. Serve with some vegetables and a sauce if you like.

Pork with Tomato & Olives

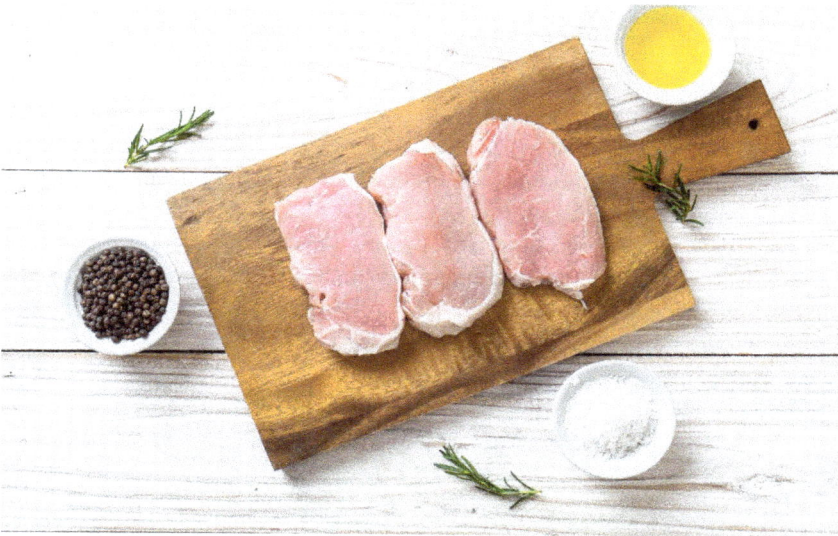

Preparation Time: 10 Minutes
Cooking Time: 30 Minutes
Servings: 6
Nutrition:
Calories 321
Fat 23 g
Carbohydrates 7 g
Protein 19 g

Ingredients:

- 6 pork chops, boneless and cut into thick slices
- 1/8 teaspoon ground cinnamon
- 1/2 cup olives, pitted and sliced
- 8 oz can tomato, crushed
- 1/4 cup beef broth
- 2 garlic cloves, chopped
- 1 large onion, sliced
- 1 tablespoon olive oil

Directions:

1. Warm up olive oil in a pan over medium heat.
2. Place pork chops in a pan and cook until lightly brown and set aside.
3. Cook garlic and onion in the same pan over medium heat, until onion is softened.
4. Add broth and bring to boil over high heat.
5. Return pork to pan and stir in crushed tomatoes and remaining ingredients.
6. Cover and simmer for 20 minutes.

Jalapeno Lamb Patties

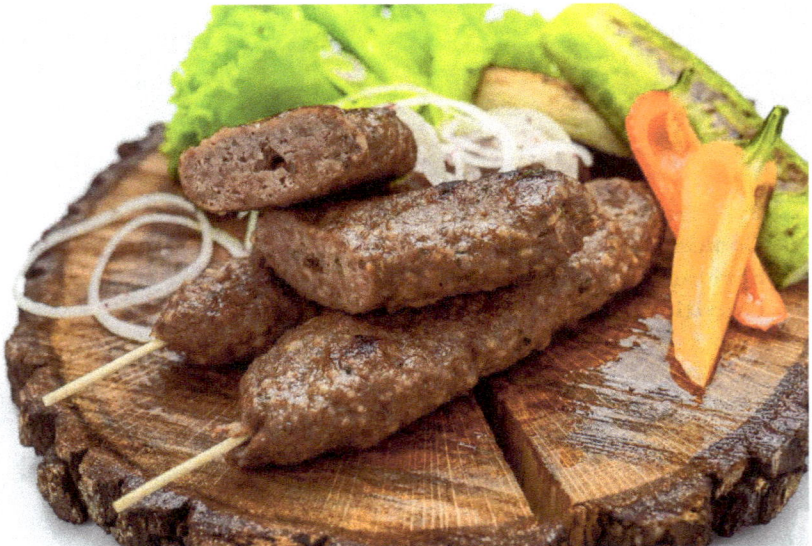

Preparation Time: 10 Minutes
Cooking Time: 8 Minutes
Servings: 4
Nutrition:
Calories 317
Fat 16 g
Carbohydrates 3 g
Protein 37.5 g

. . .

Ingredients:

- 1 lb. ground lamb
- 1 jalapeno pepper, minced
- 5 basil leaves, minced
- 10 mint leaves, minced
- ¼ cup fresh parsley, chopped
- 1 cup feta cheese, crumbled
- 1 tablespoon garlic, minced
- 1 teaspoon dried oregano
- ¼ teaspoon pepper
- ½ teaspoon kosher salt

Directions:

1. Add all fixings into the mixing bowl and mix until well combined.
2. Preheat the grill to 450 F.
3. Spray grill with cooking spray.
4. Make four equal shape patties from meat mixture and place on hot grill and cook for 3 minutes. Turn patties to another side and cook for 4 minutes.

Red Pepper Pork Tenderloin

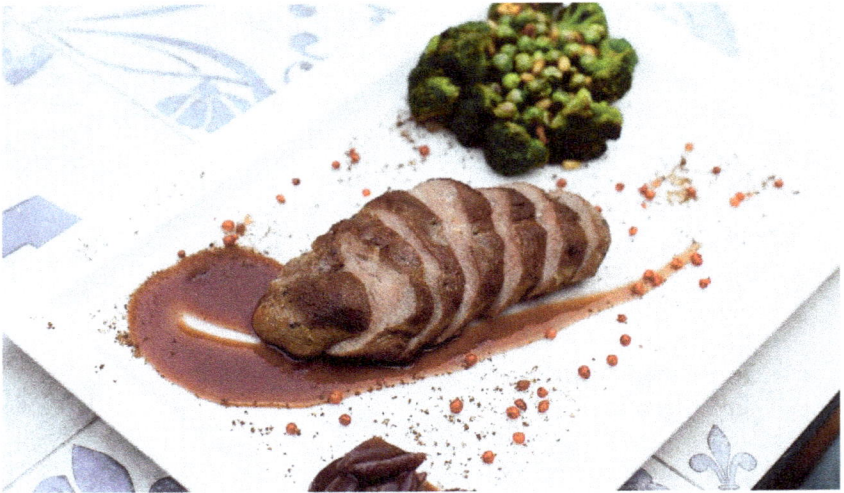

Preparation Time: 10 Minutes
Cooking Time: 25 Minutes
Servings: 4
Nutrition:
Calories 215
Fat 9.1 g
Carbohydrates 1 g
Protein 30.8 g

Ingredients:

- 1 lb. pork tenderloin
- 3/4 teaspoon red pepper
- 2 teaspoon dried oregano
- 1 tablespoon olive oil
- 3 tablespoon feta cheese, crumbled
- 3 tablespoon olive tapenades

Directions:

1. Add pork, oil, red pepper, and oregano in a zip-lock bag and rub well and place in a refrigerator for 2 hours.
2. Remove pork from zip-lock bag. Using sharp knife make lengthwise cut through the center of the tenderloin.
3. Spread olive tapenade on half tenderloin and sprinkle with feta cheese.
4. Fold another half of meat over to the original shape of tenderloin.
5. Tie close pork tenderloin with twine at 2-inch intervals.
6. Grill the pork tenderloin for 20 minutes.
7. Cut into slices and serve with some vegetables.

Basil Parmesan Pork Roast

Preparation Time: 10 Minutes
Cooking Time: 2 Hours
Servings: 8
Nutrition:
Calories 294
Fat 11.6 g
Carbohydrates 5 g
Protein 38 g
Ingredients:

- 2 lbs. lean pork roast, boneless
- 1 tablespoon parsley
- ½ cup parmesan cheese, grated
- 28 oz can tomato, diced
- 1 teaspoon dried oregano
- 1 teaspoon dried basil
- 1 teaspoon garlic powder
- Pepper
- Salt

-

Directions:

1. Add the meat into the crock pot.

2. Mix together tomatoes, oregano, basil, garlic powder, parsley, cheese, pepper, and salt and pour over meat.
3. Cook on low for 6 hours.

Sun-dried Tomato Chuck Roast

Preparation Time: 10 Minutes
Cooking Time: 2 Hours
Servings: 6
Nutrition:
Calories 582
Fat 43 g
Carbohydrates 5 g
Protein 40g
Ingredients:

- 2 lbs. beef chuck roast
- ½ cup beef broth
- ¼ cup sun-dried tomatoes, chopped
- 25 garlic cloves, peeled
- ¼ cup olives, sliced
- 1 teaspoon dried Italian seasoning, crushed
- 2 tablespoon balsamic vinegar

Directions:

1. Place meat into a pot.
2. Pour remaining ingredients over meat.
3. Cover then cook on low flame for 2 hours.
4. Shred the meat using fork.

Lamb Stew

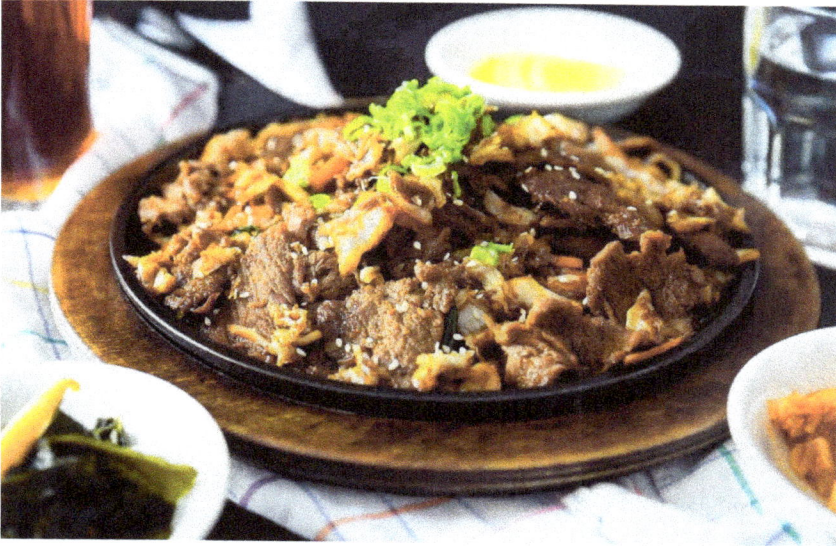

Preparation Time: 10 Minutes
Cooking Time: 3 Hours
Servings: 2
Nutrition:
Calories 297
Fat 20.3 g
Carbohydrates 5.4 g
Protein 21 g

Ingredients:

- 1/2 lb. lamb, boneless
- 1/4 cup green olives, sliced
- 2 tablespoon lemon juice
- 1/2 onion, chopped
- 2 garlic cloves, minced
- 2 fresh thyme sprigs
- 1/4 teaspoon turmeric
- 1/2 teaspoon pepper
- 1/4 Teaspoon salt
- 1/2 teaspoon sesame seeds

Directions:

1. Slice the lamb into thin pieces.
2. Add every ingredient into a pot and stir.
3. Cover and cook on low flame for 3 hours.
4. Stir well, garnish with sesame seeds and serve.

Lemon Lamb Leg

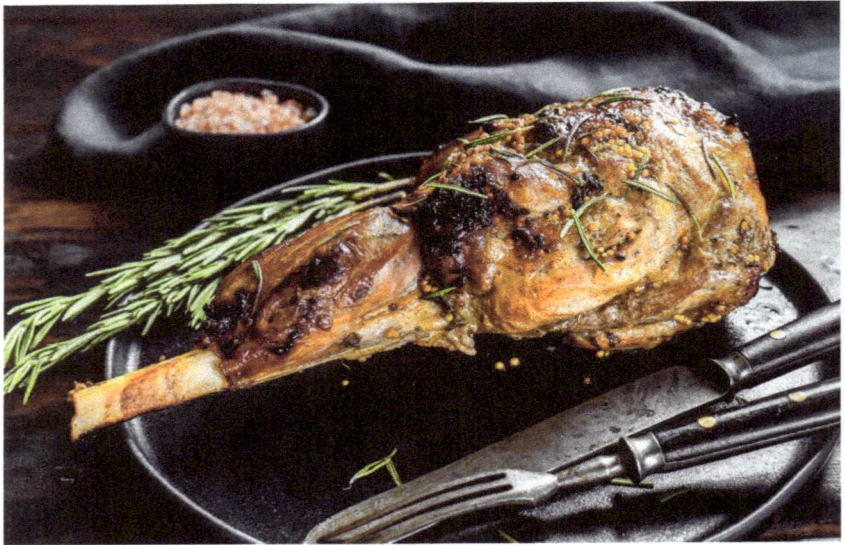

Preparation Time: 10 Minutes
Cooking Time: 2 Hours
Servings: 8

Nutrition:
Calories 275
Fat 10.2 g
Carbohydrates 0.4 g
Protein 42 g
Ingredients:

- 4 lbs. lamb leg, boneless and slice of fat
- 1 tablespoon rosemary, crushed
- 1/4 cup water
- 1/4 cup lemon juice
- 1 teaspoon black pepper
- 1/4 teaspoon salt

Directions:

1. Place lamb into a pot.
2. Add remaining ingredients over the lamb, into the pot.
3. Cover then cook on low flame for 2 hours.
4. Remove lamb from the pot and slice it.
5. Serve and enjoy.

7

Dinner

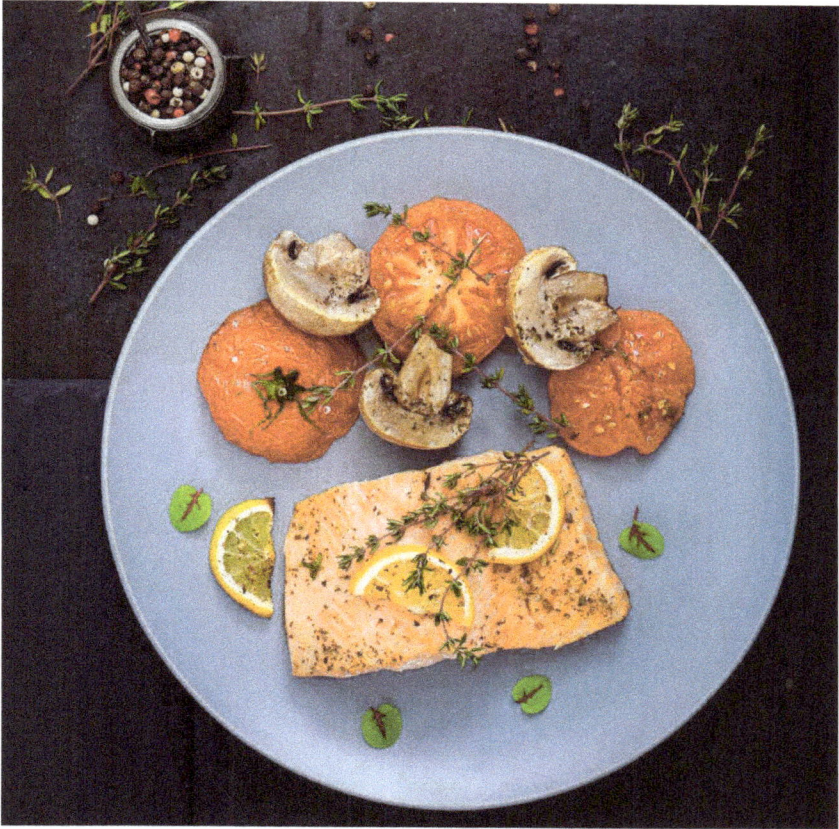

Garlic Shrimp with Olive Oil

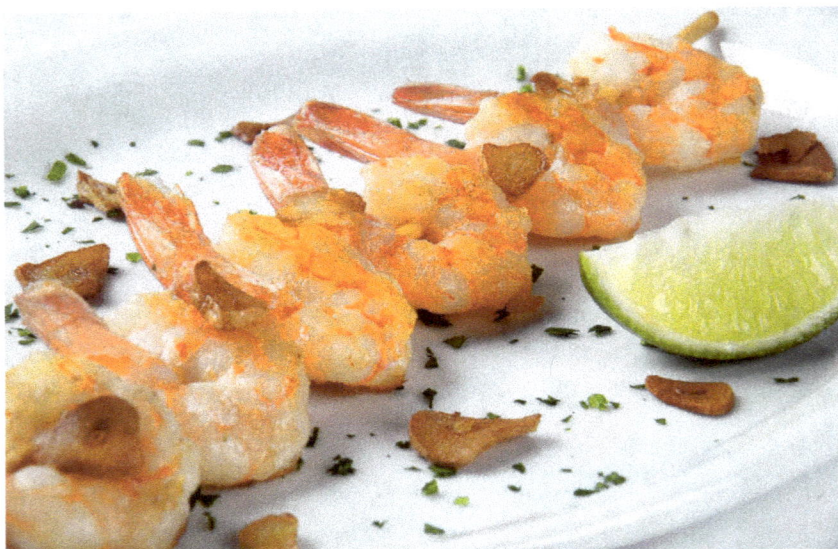

Preparation Time: 4 Minutes
Cooking Time: 10 Minutes
Servings: 5

Nutrition:
Calories:175,
Fat:2.2g,
Protein:32g,
Carbohydrate:8.3g,
Cholesterol:80mg
Ingredients:

- 1 cup extra-virgin oil
- 4 garlic cloves, minced
- 6 whole dried red chilies
- ¼ cup minced flat-leaf parsley
- 2 pounds shelled and deveined medium shrimp
- Pinch of salt
- Crusty bread, for serving (optional)

Directions:

1. Warmth olive oil in a large deep skillet until shimmering.
2. Then, add the garlic, chilies, and parsley and cook over moderately high heat for 10 seconds, stirring.
3. Add on the shrimp and cook over high heat, stirring once, until they are pink and curled 3 to 4 minutes.
4. Season with salt and pepper to taste. Transfer to small bowls.

Steamed Mussels in Tomato Garlic

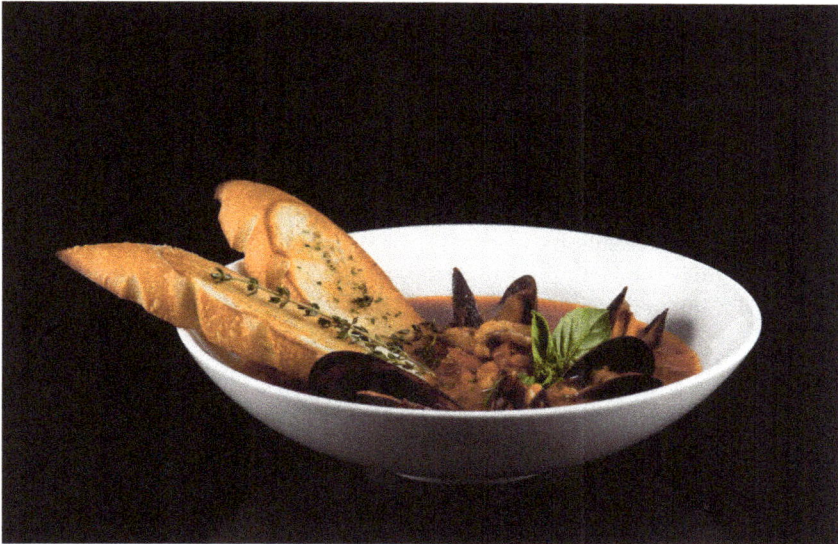

Preparation Time: 5 Minutes
Cooking Time: 23 Minutes
Servings: 4
Nutrition:
Calories:272,
Fat:5.2g,
Protein:35g,
Carbohydrate:12.7g,
Cholesterol:25mg

Ingredients:

- ¼ cup olive oil

- 1 medium-size onion, finely chopped
- 6 cloves garlic, minced
- 3 tablespoons fresh scallions, chopped
- 2 cups canned tomatoes, chopped
- ¼ teaspoon dried thyme
- ¼ teaspoon dried red-pepper flakes
- 4 pounds' mussels, cleaned
- 1/8 teaspoon freshly ground black pepper
- Pinch of salt to taste
- Crusty bread (optional)

Directions:

1. Prepare a large pot, then heat the oil over moderately low heat.
2. Then put the onion and garlic then cook, stirring occasionally, until the onion is translucent, about 5 minutes.
3. Stir in the scallions, tomatoes, thyme, and red pepper flakes.
4. Reduce the heat and simmer, partially covered, for 15 minutes, stirring occasionally.
5. Add the mussels to the pot. Cover; bring to a boil.
6. Cook, and stir the pot occasionally, just until the mussels open, about 3 minutes. Remove the open mussels.
7. Continue to boil, uncovering the pot as necessary to remove the mussels as soon as their shells open. Discard any that do not open longer.
8. Stir the black pepper into the broth. Add salt to taste.
9. Ladle the broth over the mussels. Serve with crusty bread. Enjoy!

Mediterranean-style Mussels

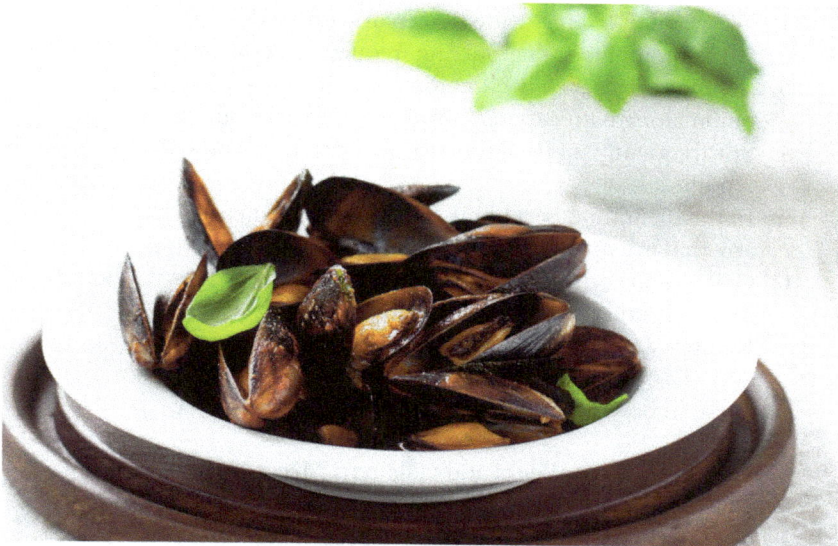

Preparation Time: 5 Minutes
Cooking Time: 21 Minutes
Servings: 2
Nutrition:
Calories:212,
Fat:8.3g,
Protein:18.2g,
Carbohydrate:11.7g,
Cholesterol:35mg

Ingredients:

- 1 medium-size onion, chopped
- 5 cloves garlic, minced
- 1 tablespoon extra-virgin olive oil
- 4 ripe tomatoes, plum
- 1 small size bell pepper
- 1 tablespoon capers, drained
- 1 teaspoon dried oregano
- 500g mussels, cleaned

Directions:

1. Warm oil in a large, wide saucepan with medium heat.
2. Add onion plus garlic. Stirring frequently, cook for 3 min.
3. Temporarily, coarsely chop tomatoes and pepper. Add to the onion along with capers. Sprinkling with seasonings.
4. Stir frequently up until tomatoes start to break down, 5 to 7 min.
5. In the meantime, scrub mussels and pull off beards. Discard any that are open. Stir into a thickened tomato mixture.
6. Cover then cook up until majority of the mussels open, about 6 min. Stir midway through cooking.
7. Remove any mussels that are not open after 6 min. Palate and add salt if desirable.
8. Serve in bowls plus crusty bread. Enjoy!

Leeks and Calamari Mix

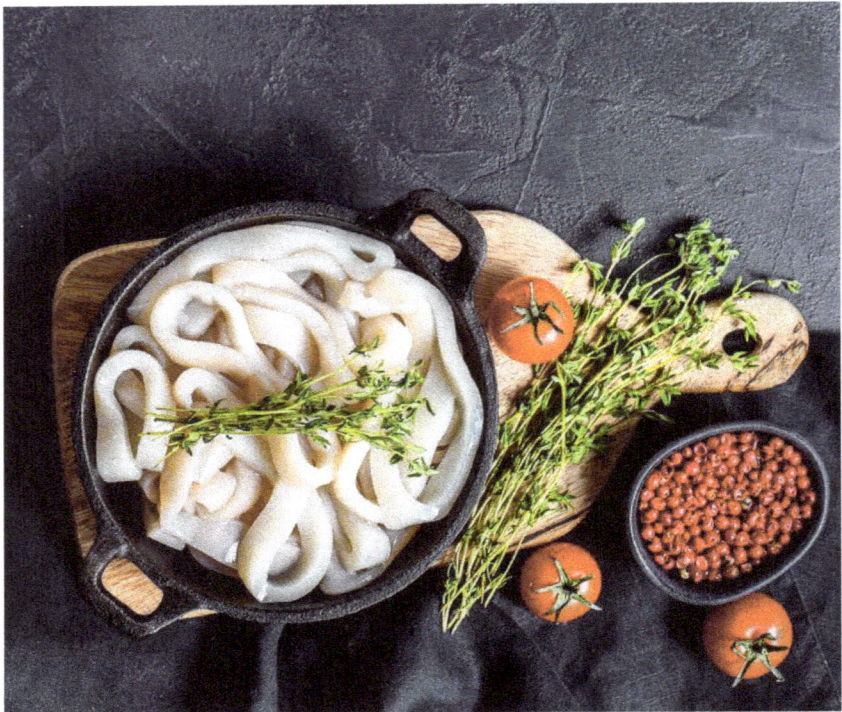

Preparation Time: 5 Minutes
Cooking Time: 15 Minutes
Servings: 4

Nutrition:
Calories:238,
Fat:9g,
Protein:8.4g,
Carbohydrate:14.4g,
Cholesterol:95mg

Ingredients:

- 2 tablespoons avocado oil
- 2 leeks, chopped
- 1 red onion, chopped
- Salt and black to the taste
- 1-pound calamari rings
- 1 tablespoon parsley, chopped
- 1 tablespoon chives, chopped
- 2 tablespoons tomato paste

Directions:

1. Heat a pan with the avocado oil over medium heat, add the leeks and the onion, stir and sauté for 5 minutes.
2. Add the rest of the ingredients, toss, simmer over medium heat for 10 minutes, divide into bowls and serve.

Seafood Paella

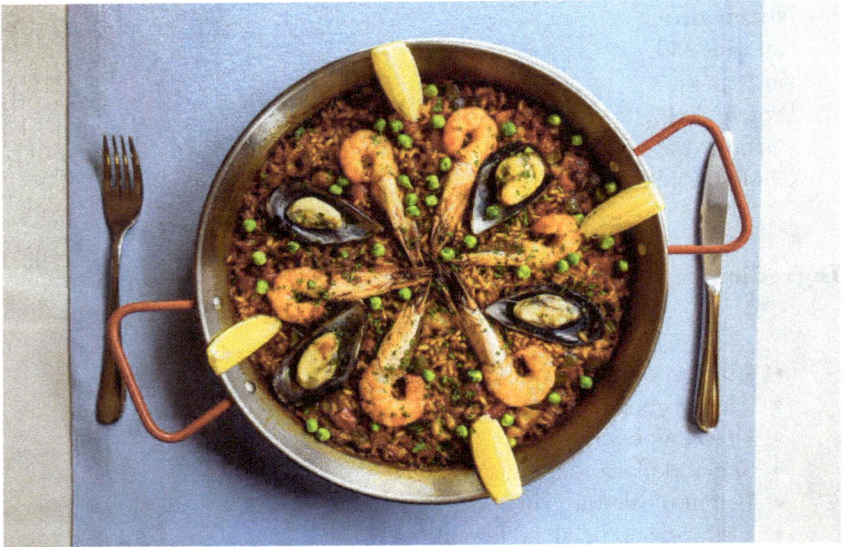

Preparation Time: 5 Minutes
Cooking Time: 35 Minutes
Servings: 4
Nutrition:
Calories:233,
Fat:5.2g,
Protein:13g,
Carbohydrate:33g,
Cholesterol:18mg

Ingredients:

- 1 tablespoon extra-virgin olive oil
- 4 cloves garlic, minced
- 1 medium-size onion, finely chopped
- 1 red bell pepper, finely chopped
- 300g short or medium grain rice
- ½ teaspoon turmeric
- 1 teaspoon paprika
- 1 14-ounces canned tomatoes, chopped
- 3 cups chicken stock
- 2 pinches of saffron threads

- 12 large shrimp, peeled and deveined
- 12 little neck mussels, thawed
- Handful fresh parsley, roughly chopped
- Lemon wedges

Directions:

1. In a deep pan with medium-high heat, add olive oil, garlic, onion, and red bell pepper and cook for 3 minutes or until vegetables softened.
2. Then, add rice, turmeric, and paprika and stir well. Then add tomatoes, chicken stock and saffron, stir and bring to a boil.
3. Lower heat to simmer and cover and cook for another 20 minutes. Spread shrimp, mussels, and green peas on top.
4. Cover then cook for additional 10-15 minutes, until mussels have opened and shrimps are pink.
5. Turn off the heat and sprinkle with parsley on top. Serve with lemon wedges on top. Enjoy!

Baked Salmon in Garlic Pepper

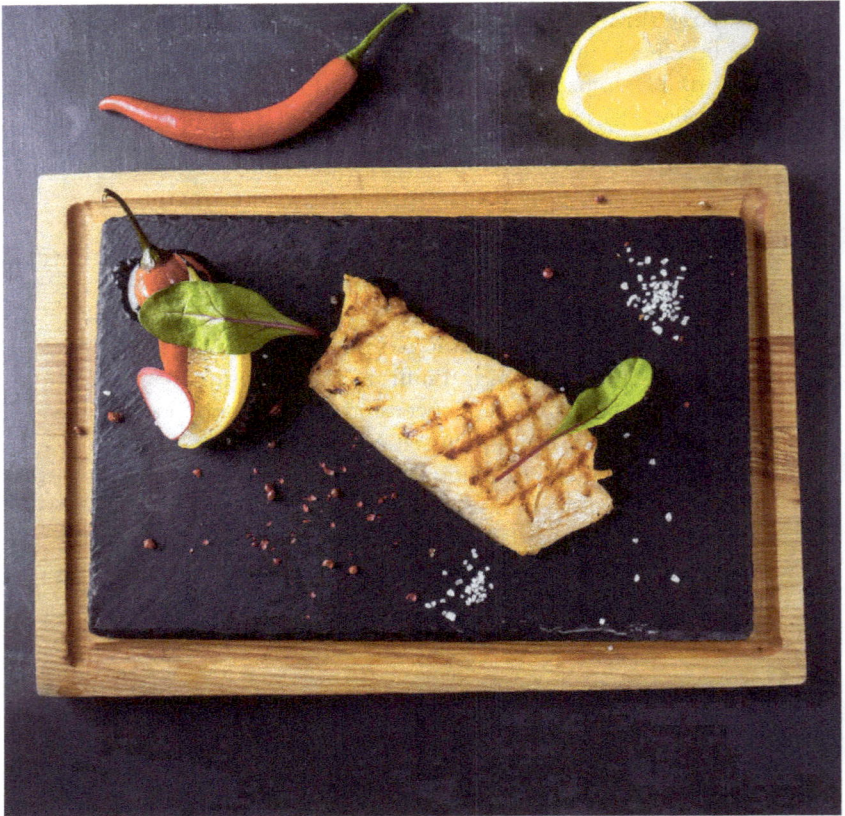

Preparation Time: 10 Minutes
Cooking Time: 25 Minutes
Servings: 3
Nutrition:
Calories:294,
Fat:11.3g,
Protein:28.2g,
Carbohydrate:1.7g,
Cholesterol:85mg

Ingredients:

- 4 (6-ounce) salmon fillets

- 4 tablespoons unsalted butter
- 1 tablespoon garlic, minced
- 3 tablespoons capers, drained
- Fresh herbs like parsley, chives or dill
- Salt and Pepper
- Lemon quartered

Directions:

1. Heat the oven to 325 degrees Fahrenheit. Season each sides of the salmon thru salt and pepper.
2. Thaw the butter in a wide oven-safe skillet over medium heat.
3. When the butter is sparkling, stirring in the garlic plus the capers. Cook, stirring, till warm, about 1 minute.
4. Take away the skillet off of the heat. Put the salmon fillets, skin-side down, to the skillet.
5. Slant the pan so that butter pools on one side then spoon garlic caper butter over each fillet.
6. Cover the frying pan with a sheet of aluminum foil or conceal with parchment paper by lightly tucking it around the salmon.
7. Bake the salmon, enclosed, for 15 minutes. Bare then spoon extra of the butter over the salmon.
8. Remain to roast, open, until your chosen doneness, 5 to 10 minutes more, depending on how thick the salmon is. Tip: We cook salmon until an instant-read thermometer reads 125 degrees Fahrenheit when inserted into the thickest part.
9. On the other hand, finish cooking the salmon with the broiler for some additional color on top. Watch thoroughly so the fish does not burn.
10. Squash fresh lemon juice over the baked salmon, sprinkle with lots of fresh herbs.
11. Serve with additional spoonful of the garlic caper butter on top. Enjoy!

Sauteed Octopus

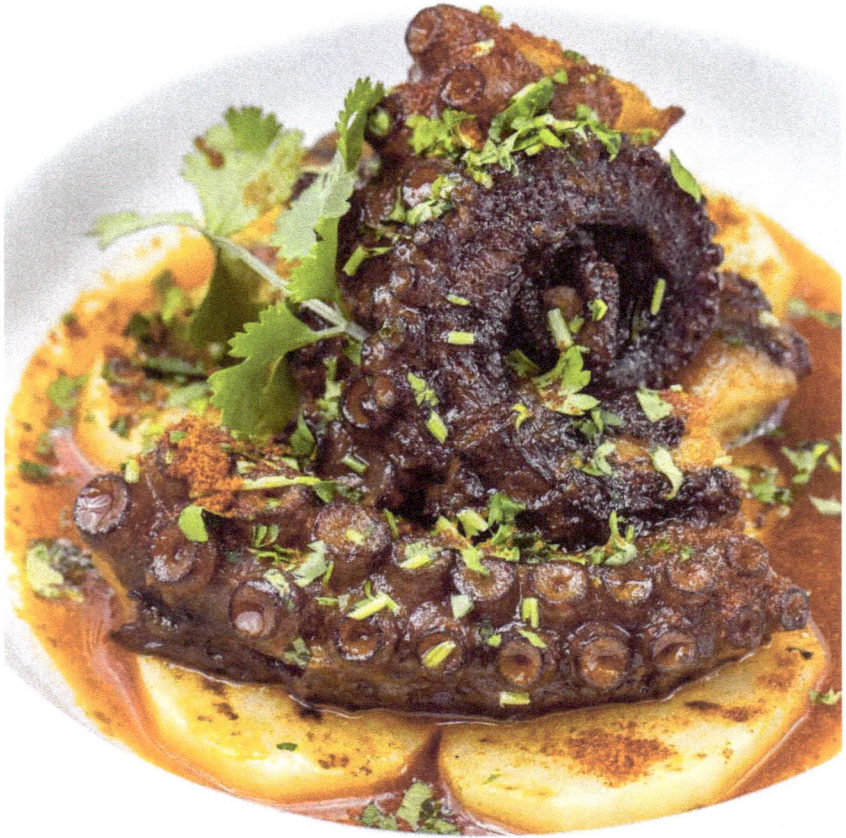

Preparation Time: 5 Minutes
Cooking Time: 1 Hour 10 Minutes
Servings: 4

Nutrition:
Calories:274,
Fat:8.3g,
Protein:35.2g,

Carbohydrate:9.8g,
Cholesterol:75mg

Ingredients:

- 2 pounds' whole octopus, cleaned and cooked ahead (see the Directions below)
- 2 tablespoons extra-virgin olive oil
- 2 medium-size green chili
- 2 plum tomatoes, sliced
- ¼ pitted olives
- 2 tablespoons fresh oregano leaves, chopped
- 2 teaspoons cider vinegar

Directions:

How to cook the whole octopus:

1. All frozen octopus is pre-cleaned, and if buying fresh, you can ask the fishmonger to clean it for you.
2. In a large pot, let water to boil and then diminish to a simmer. Put the whole octopus, and simmer for 1 hour.
3. Take away the octopus from boiling water, and let cool at room temperature for 15 minutes.
4. To Sauté: Cut the tentacles from the head, and discard the head. Chop the tentacles into small pieces.
5. Heat a large sauté pan with olive oil over medium heat, add the octopus, green chili, tomatoes, olives, oregano, and vinegar.
6. Sauté for 10 minutes. Serve immediately.

Grilled Octopus

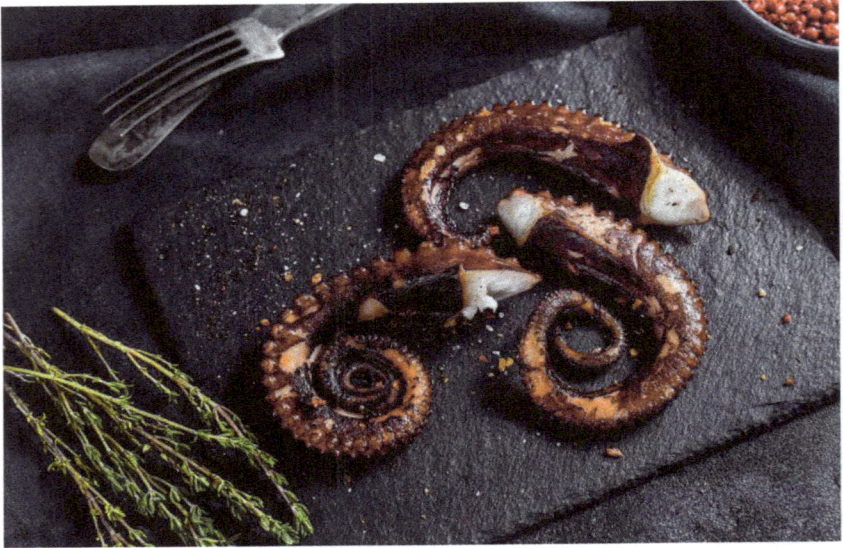

Preparation Time: 40 Minutes
Cooking Time: 1 Hour 15 Minutes
Servings: 4

Nutrition:
Calories:243,
Fat:6.3g,
Protein:38.2g,
Carbohydrate:4g,
Cholesterol:0mg

Ingredients:

- 1 pound of fresh octopus (medium or large), cleaned and cook ahead
- 1/3 cup freshly squeezed lemon juice
- ¼ cup lemon zest
- 2 garlic heads, minced
- 2 tablespoon parsley, minced
- ½ teaspoon dried oregano
- 2/3 cup Olive oil

- Salt and Pepper, to taste

Directions:

1. Arrange octopus in a pot then cover with enough water. Bring to boil for 40 minutes.
2. Remove the octopus from hot water, rinse it then transfer it in a bowl.
3. Drizzle with olive oil plus the chopped garlic. Let it cool for 30 minutes to 1 hour.
4. Preheat a gas grill to medium-high heat. Slice octopus's tentacles.
5. Grill for 3 or 4 minutes each side until charred. Take away from heat then put it in a bowl.
6. Drizzle with olive oil then add lemon juice. Put salt and pepper.
7. Sprinkle some oregano and parsley on top. Add some garlic (optional).

Scallop Salad

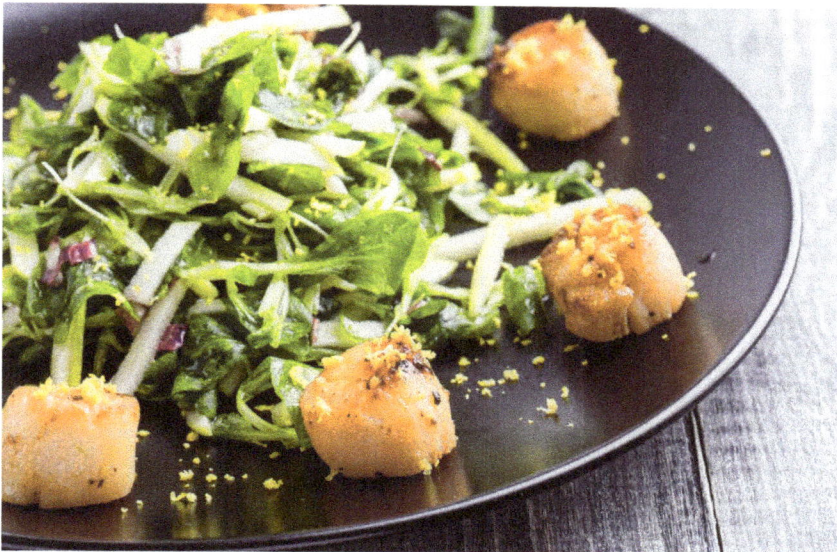

Preparation Time: 15 Minutes
Cooking Time: 35 Minutes
Servings: 6
Nutrition:

Calories:201,
Fat:5g,
Fiber:2g,
Carbs:5g,
Protein:8g

Ingredients:

- 12 ounces dry sea scallops
- 4 tablespoons olive oil + 2 teaspoons
- 4 teaspoons soy sauce
- 1 ½ cup quinoa, rinsed
- 2 teaspoons garlic, minced
- A pinch of salt
- 3 cups water
- 1 cup snow peas, sliced
- 1 teaspoon sesame oil
- 1/3 cup rice vinegar
- 1 cup scallions, sliced
- 1/3 cup red bell pepper, chopped
- ¼ cup cilantro, chopped

Directions:

1. In a bowl, mix scallops with 2 teaspoons soy sauce, toss and leave aside for now.
2. Warmth a pan with 1 tablespoon olive oil over medium heat, add quinoa, stir and cook for 8 minutes. Add garlic, stir and cook for 1 more minute.
3. Add water and a pinch of salt, bring to a boil, stir, cover and cook for 15 minutes. Add snow peas, cover and leave for 5 more minutes.
4. Meanwhile, in a bowl, mix 3 tablespoons olive oil with 2 teaspoons soy sauce, vinegar and sesame oil and whisk well.
5. Add quinoa and snow peas to mixture and stir again. Add scallions, bell pepper and stir again.
6. Pat dry the scallions and discard marinade. Heat another pan with 2 teaspoons olive oil over medium high heat, add scallions and cook for 1 minute on each side.

7. Add scallops to quinoa salad, stir gently and serve with chopped cilantro on top.

Delicious Chicken Soup

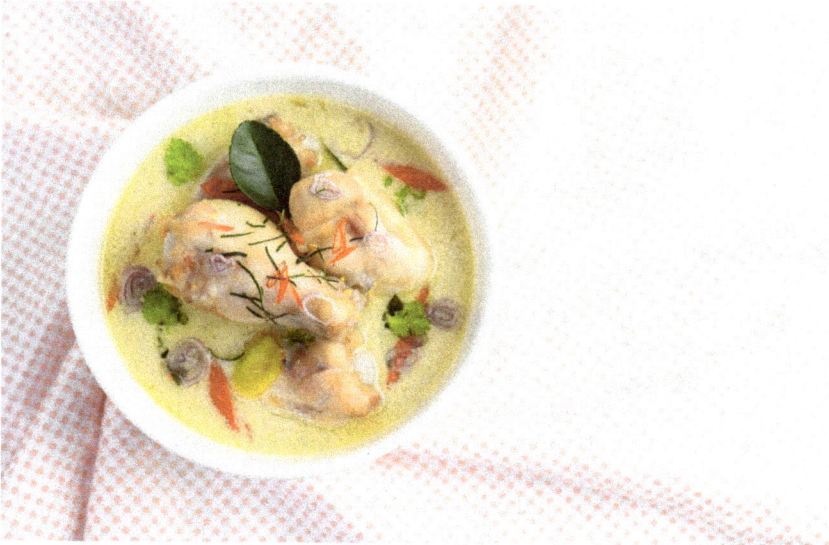

Preparation Time: 10 Minutes
Cooking Time: 1 Hour
Servings: 8

Nutrition:
Calories:242,
Fat:3g,
Fiber:2g,
Carbs:5g,
Protein:3g
Ingredients:

- 2 cups eggplant, diced
- Salt and black pepper to taste
- ¼ cup olive oil + 1 tablespoon cup yellow
- onion, chopped
- tablespoons garlic, minced

- red bell pepper, chopped
- hot paprika 2 + teaspoons
- ¼ cup parsley, chopped
- teaspoon turmeric
- and ½ tablespoons oregano, chopped
- cups chicken stock pound chicken breast, skinless, boneless and cut into small pieces c
- up half and half and ½ tablespoons cornstarch
- egg yolks
- ¼ cup lemon juice
- Lemon wedges for serving

Directions:

1. In a bowl, mix eggplant pieces with ¼ cup oil, salt and pepper to taste and toss to coat.
2. Arrange eggplant on a lined baking sheet, place in the oven at 400 degrees F and bake for 10 minutes.
3. Flip, cook for 10 minutes more and set aside to cool. Heat a saucepan with 1 tablespoon oil over medium heat, add garlic and onion, cover and cook for 10 minutes.
4. Add bell pepper, stir and cook uncovered for 3 minutes. Add hot paprika, ginger and turmeric and stir well. Add the stock, chicken, eggplant pieces, oregano and parsley.
5. Stir, bring to a boil and simmer for 12 minutes. In a bowl, mix cornstarch with half and half and egg yolks - stir well.

6. Add 1 cup soup, stir again and pour gradually into soup. Stir then put salt and pepper to taste and lemon juice. Ladle into soup bowls and serve with lemon wedges on the side.

Classic Mediterranean Chicken Soup

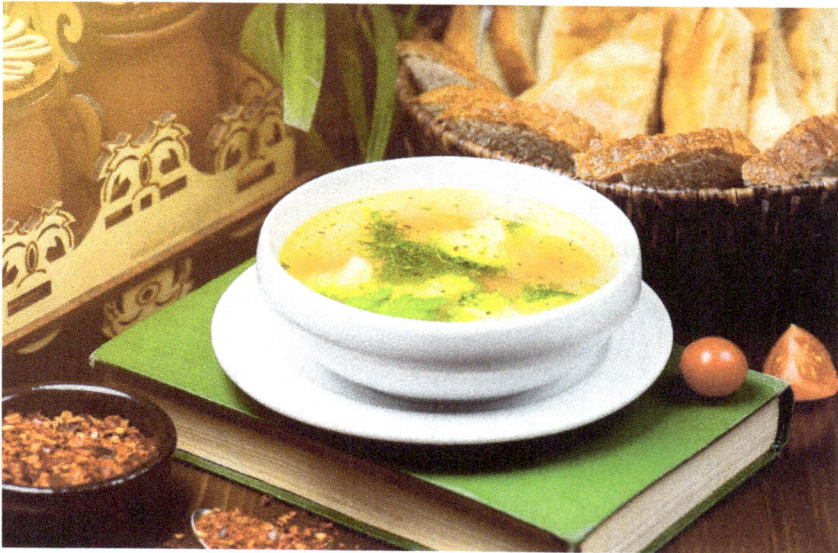

Preparation Time: 15 Minutes
Cooking Time: 1 Hour 20 Minutes
Servings: 4
Nutrition:
Calories:242,
Fat:3g,
Fiber:2g,
Carbs:3g,
Protein:3g

Ingredients:

- big chicken
- tablespoons salt
- cups water leak, cut in quarters
- bay leaves carrot, cut into quarters
- tablespoons olive oil
- 2/3 cup rice
- cups yellow onion, chopped
- eggs ½ cup lemon juice
- teaspoon
- black pepper

Directions:

1. Put chicken in a large saucepan, add water and 2 tablespoons salt, bring to a boil over medium high heat, reduce heat and skim foam.
2. Add carrot, bay leaves and leek and simmer for 1 hour. Heat a pan with the oil over medium high heat, add onion, stir and cook for 6 minutes, take off heat and leave aside for now.
3. Transfer chicken to a cutting board and leave aside to cool down. Strain soup back into the saucepan.
4. Add sautéed onion and rice, bring again to a boil over high heat, reduce temperature to low and simmer for 20 minutes.
5. Discard chicken bones and skin, dice into big chunks and return to boiling soup. Meanwhile, in a bowl, mix lemon juice with eggs and black pepper and stir well.
6. Add 2 cups boiling soup and whisk again well.
7. Pour this into the soup and stir well.
8. Add remaining salt, stir, take off heat, transfer to soup bowls and serve right away.

Easy Chicken Stew

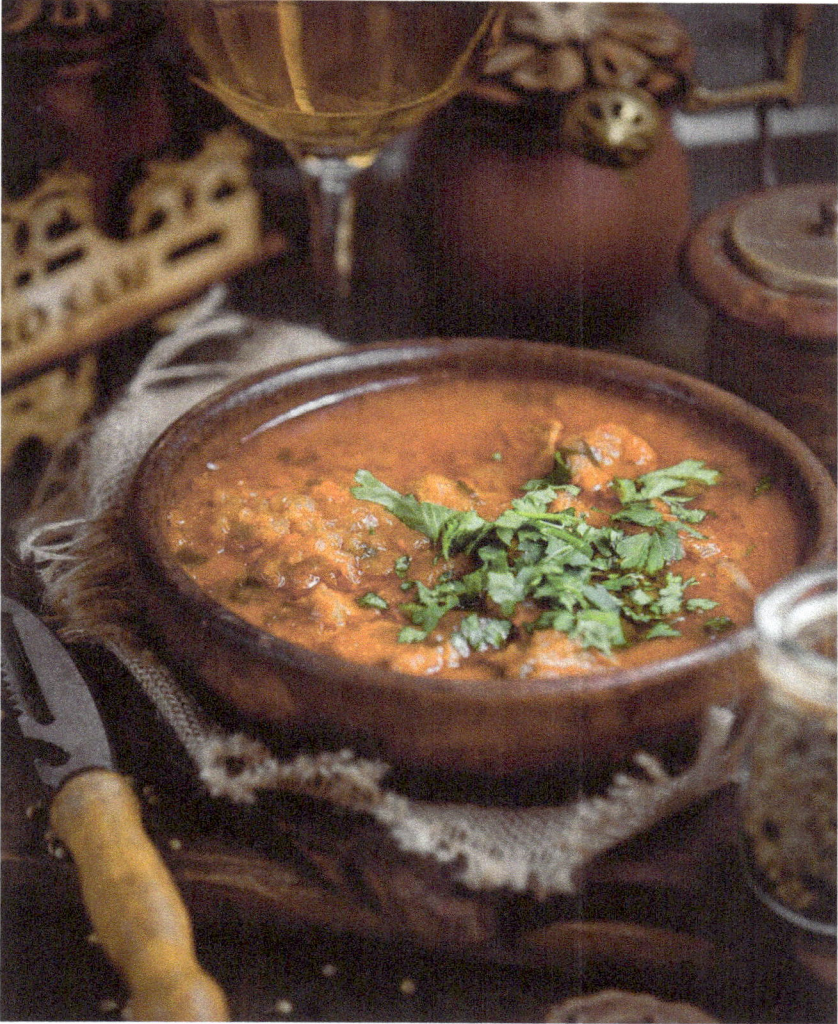

Preparation Time: 20 Minutes
Cooking Time: 40 Minutes
Servings: 4

Nutrition:
Calories:200,
Fat:4g,
Fiber:3g,

Carbs:7g,
Protein:12g
Ingredients:

- 3 ½ pounds chicken, cut into 10 medium pieces
- 2 yellow onions, chopped
- 2 tablespoons olive oil garlic clove, minced
- ¼ pint chicken stock, warm tablespoon white flour
- teaspoons mixed dried herbs (parsley and basil)
- 14 ounces canned tomatoes, chopped
- Salt and black pepper to taste

Directions:

1. Heat a saucepan with the oil over medium high heat, add chicken meat, stir and brown it for 5 minutes, take off heat, transfer to a plate and set aside.
2. Return saucepan to heat, add garlic and onion, stir and cook for 3 minutes.
3. Add flour and stir well. Add herbs, tomatoes and stock, stir, bring to a boil and season with salt and pepper to taste.
4. Add chicken pieces, stir, reduce heat to medium and simmer the stew for 45 minutes. Transfer to plates and serve right away.

Chicken and Cabbage Mix

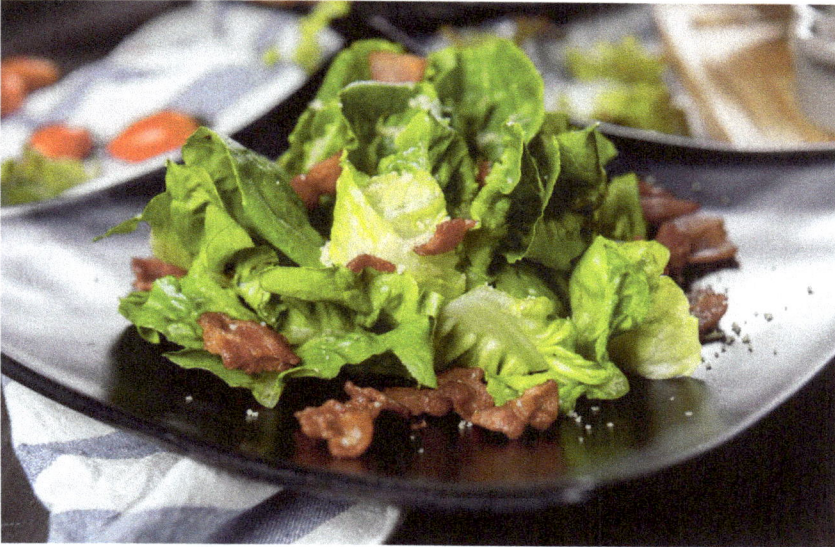

Preparation Time: 10 Minutes
Cooking Time: 6 Minutes
Servings: 4

Nutrition:
Calories:200,
Fat:15g,
Fiber:3g,
Carbs:10g,
Protein:33g

Ingredients:

- 3 medium chicken breasts, skinless, boneless and cut into thin strips
- 4 ounces green cabbage, shredded
- 5 tablespoon extra-virgin olive oil
- Salt and black pepper to taste
- 2 tablespoons sherry vinegar tablespoon chives, chopped
- ¼ cup feta cheese, crumbled
- ¼ cup barbeque sauce

- bacon slices, cooked and crumbled

Directions:

1. In a bowl, mix 4 tablespoon oil with vinegar, salt and pepper to taste and stir well.
2. Add the shredded cabbage, toss to coat and leave aside for now.
3. Season chicken with salt and pepper, heat a pan with remaining oil over medium high heat, add chicken, cook for 6 minutes, take off heat, transfer to a bowl and mix well with barbeque sauce.
4. Arrange salad on serving plates, add chicken strips, sprinkle cheese, chives and crumbled bacon and serve right away.

Mediterranean Chicken and Rice Soup

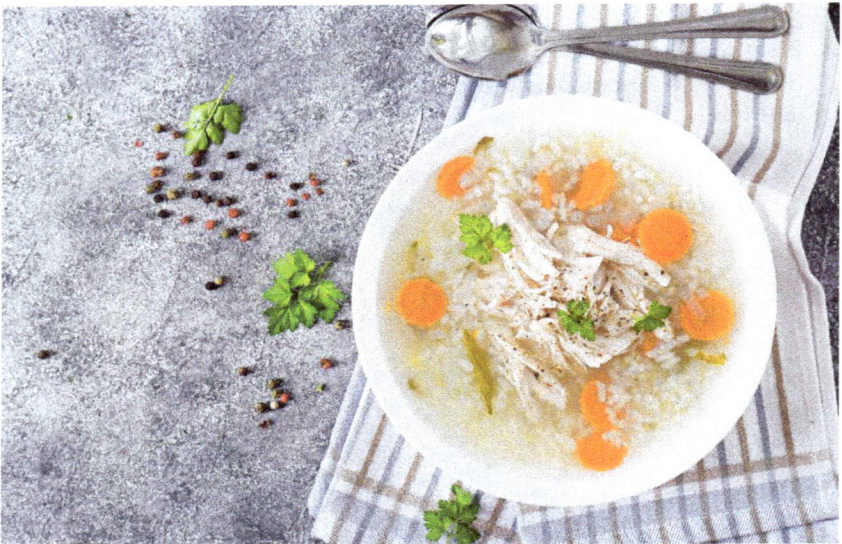

Preparation Time: 10 Minutes
Cooking Time: 40 Minutes
Servings: 8
Nutrition:
Calories:271,
Fat:5g,
Fiber:1g,

Carbs:13g,
Protein:16g

Ingredients:

- tablespoon Greek seasoning
- A pinch of salt and black pepper
- tablespoon capers
- tablespoon olive oil
- 4 spring onions, chopped
- garlic clove, minced
- teaspoons basil, chopped
- teaspoons oregano, chopped
- cup brown rice
- cups chicken stock
- ¼ cup kalamata olives, pitted and sliced
- ¼ cup sun-dried tomatoes, chopped
- tablespoons lemon juice
- teaspoons parsley, chopped
- pound chicken breast boneless, skinless and cubed

Directions:

1. Heat a saucepan with the oil over medium heat, add the chicken and brown for 2-3 minutes.
2. Add Greek seasoning, salt, pepper and the garlic, stir and cook for 3 minutes more.
3. Add the capers, spring onions, basil, oregano, rice, stock, olives, tomatoes, and lemon juice, stir, bring to a boil and simmer for 30 minutes.
4. Add the parsley, stir, ladle the soup into bowls and serve.

Healthy Mediterranean Chicken

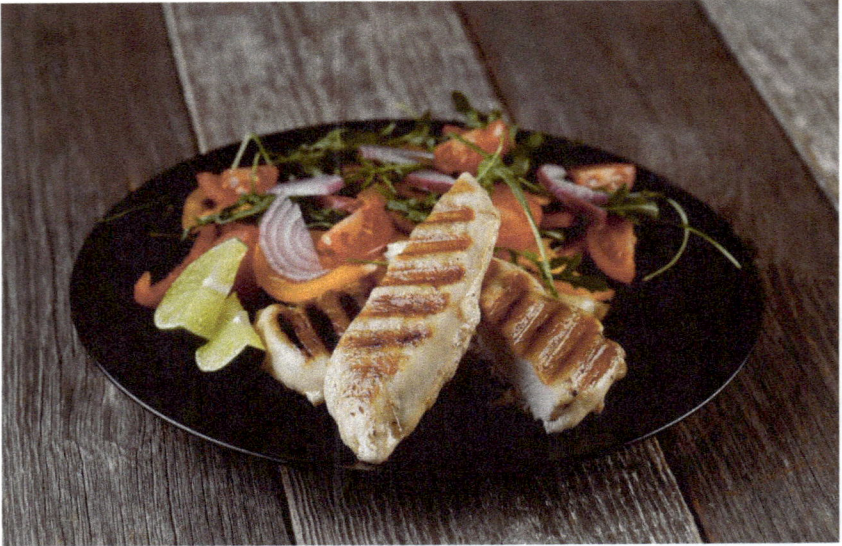

Preparation Time: 5 Minutes
Cooking Time: 6 Hours 10 Minutes
Servings: 6
Nutrition:
Calories:342,
Fat:3g,
Fiber:3g,
Carbs:5g,
Protein:4g

Ingredients:

- 2 pounds chicken breasts, boneless and skinless
- 28 ounces canned tomatoes, chopped
- 28 ounces canned artichoke hearts, drained
- ½ cups chicken stock yellow onion, chopped
- ¼ cup white wine vinegar
- ½ cup kalamata olives, pitted and chopped
- tablespoon curry powder
- teaspoons thyme
- teaspoons basil
- Salt and black pepper to taste

- ¼ cup parsley, chopped

Directions:

1. Put chicken breasts in a slow cooker.
2. Add tomatoes, artichoke hearts, onion and olives and stir.
3. Add stock, vinegar, curry powder, thyme, basil, salt and black pepper to taste.
4. Close the lid then cook on Low for 6 hours. Uncover, add more salt and pepper if needed, add parsley and stir gently.

Mushroom and Chicken Bowl

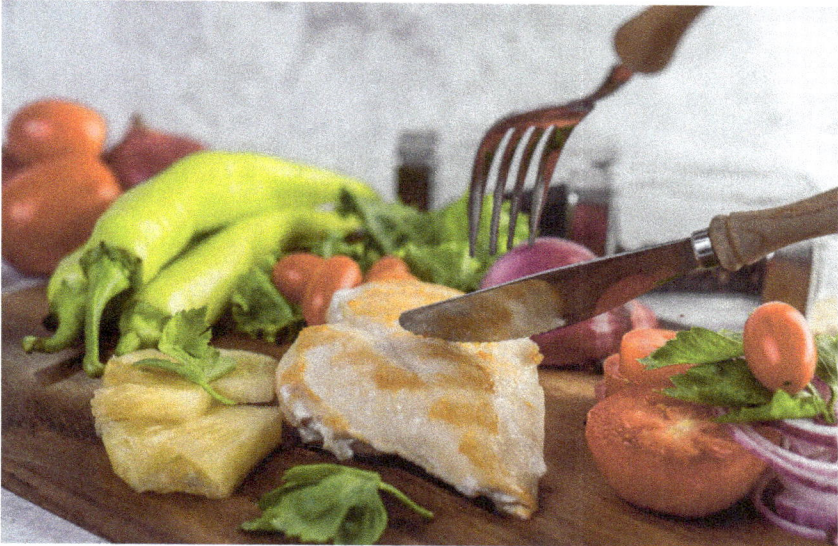

Preparation Time: 10 Minutes
Cooking Time: 25 Minutes
Servings: 4
Nutrition:
Calories:200,
Fat:15g,
Fiber:3g,
Carbs:10g,
Protein:33g

. . .

Ingredients:

- 1 and ½ cups unsweetened coconut milk
- 1-pound chicken thigh, skinless
- 3-4 garlic cloves, crushed
- ½ an onion, finely diced
- 2-inch knob ginger, minced
- 1 cup mushrooms, sliced
- 4 ounces baby spinach
- ½ teaspoon of cayenne pepper
- ½ teaspoon turmeric
- 1 teaspoon salt
- 1 teaspoon Garam Masala
- ¼ cup cilantro, chopped

Directions:

1. Add the listed ingredients to your Ninja Foodi
2. Close and cook on HIGH pressure for 15 minutes
3. Release pressure naturally over 10 minutes
4. Remove chicken and roughly puree the veggies using an immersion blender
5. Shred chicken and add it back to the pot. Add cream and stir. Serve and enjoy!

Chicken and Broccoli Platter

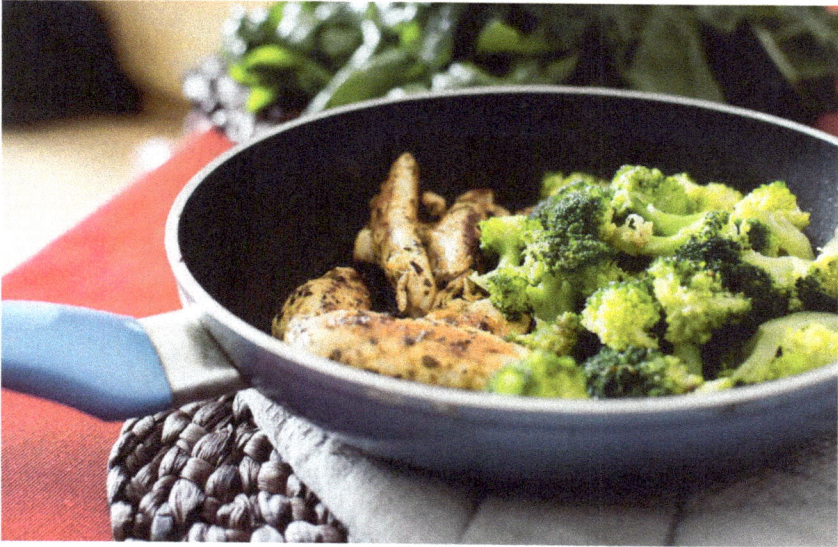

Preparation Time: 10 Minutes
Cooking Time: 20 Minutes
Servings: 4
Nutrition:
Calories:230,
Fat:12g,
Fiber:12g,
Carbs:34g,
Protein:13g

Ingredients:

- 1 tablespoon olive oil
- 1 tablespoon butter
- 2 large chicken breasts, boneless
- ½ cup onion, chopped
- 14 ounces chicken broth
- ½ teaspoon salt
- ½ teaspoon pepper
- 1/8 teaspoon red pepper flakes
- 1 tablespoon parsley
- 1 tablespoon arrowroot

- 2 tablespoons water
- 4 ounces light cream cheese, cubed
- 1 cup cheddar cheese, shredded
- 3 cups steamed broccoli, chopped

Directions:

1. Put pepper and salt in the chicken breast
2. Set your Ninja Foodi to Sauté mode and add butter and vegetable oil
3. Allow it to melt and transfer the seasoned chicken to the pot. Allow it to brown
4. Remove the chicken and add the onions to the pot, Sauté them for 5 minutes
5. Add chicken broth, pepper, red pepper and salt, parsley. Add the browned breast
6. Lock up the lid and cook for about 5 minutes at high pressure
7. Once done, quick release the pressure. Remove the chicken and shred it up into small portions
8. Take a bowl and add 2 tablespoons of water and dissolve cornstarch \
9. Select the simmer mode and add the mixture to the Ninja Foodi
10. Toss in the cubed and shredded cheese. Stir completely until everything is melted
11. Toss in the diced chicken again and the steamed broccoli and cook for 5 minutes
12. Once done, sever with white rice and shredded cheese as garnish.

Daring Salted Baked Chicken

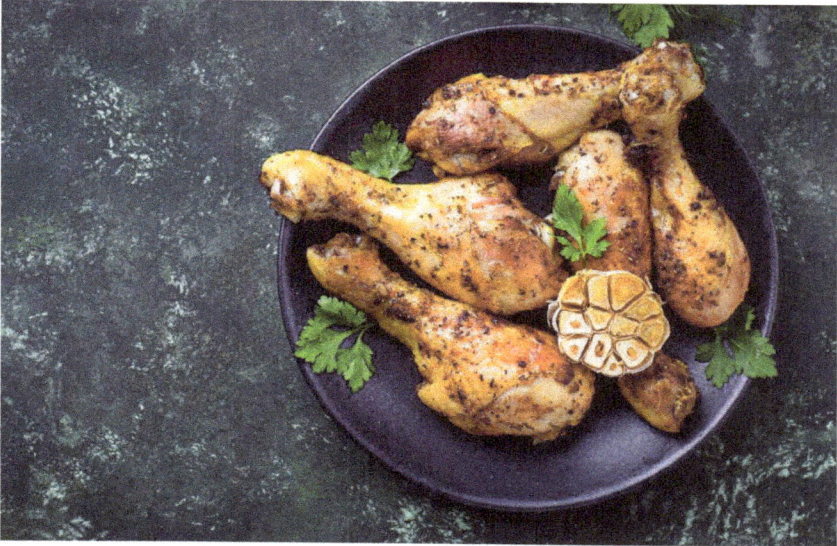

Preparation Time: 10 Minutes
Cooking Time: 26 Minutes
Servings: 6
Nutrition:
Calories:145,
Fat:4g,
Fiber:3g,
Carbs:11g,
Protein:4g

Ingredients:

- 2 teaspoons ginger, minced
- 1 and ¼ teaspoons salt
- ¼ teaspoons five spice powder
- Dash of white pepper
- 5-6 chicken legs

Directions:

1. Season the chicken legs by placing them in a large mixing bowl

2. Pour 2 teaspoon of ginger, 1 and a ¼ teaspoon of kosher salt, ¼ teaspoon of five spice powder and mix
3. Transfer them to a parchment paper
4. Wrap up tightly and place them to a shallow dish
5. Place a steamer rack in your Ninja Foodi and add 1 cup of water
6. Place the chicken dish onto the rack
7. Close up the lid then cook on HIGH pressure for 18-26 minutes
8. Release the pressure naturally
9. Open the lid and unwrap the paper
10. Pour the juice into a small bowl
11. Transfer the chicken on a wire rack and broil for a while
12. Serve immediately with the cooking liquid used as a dipping sauce

Worthy Gee-licious Chicken

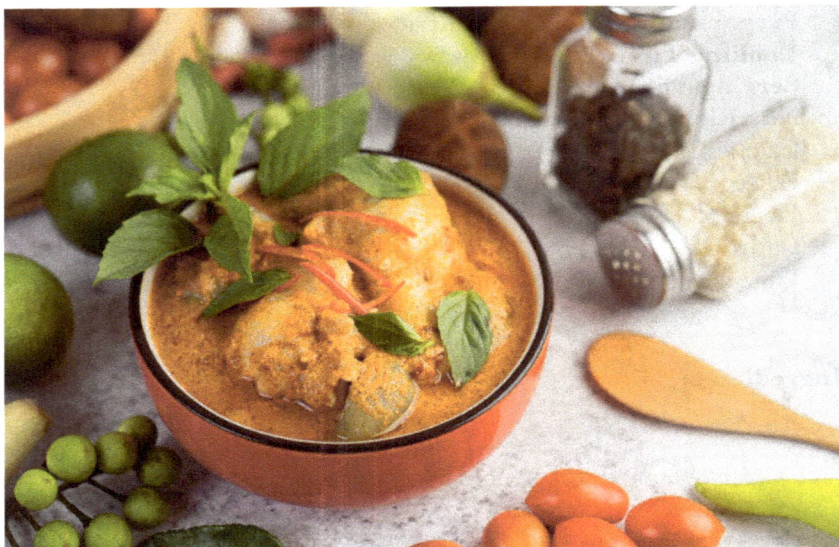

Preparation Time: 5 Minutes
Cooking Time: 10 Minutes
Servings: 6
Nutrition:
Calories:230,
Fat:12g,

Fiber:12g,
Carbs:34g,
Protein:13g

Ingredients:

- 2-3 pounds boneless chicken thigh
- 1 tablespoon ghee
- 1 and a ½ large onion, chopped
- 3 and ½ teaspoons salt
- 2 teaspoons garlic powder
- 2 teaspoons ginger powder
- 2 heaping teaspoons turmeric
- 1 and ½ teaspoon cayenne powder
- 1 and ½ cup stewed tomatoes
- 1 cup stewed tomatoes
- 2 cans of coconut milk
- 2 heaping teaspoons Garam masala
- ½ cup almond, sliced
- ½ cup cilantro

Directions:

1. Set your Ninja Foodi to Sauté mode and add ghee, allow it to melt
2. Add 2 teaspoon of salt alongside onion and cook well
3. Add ginger, garlic, turmeric, paprika, cayenne pepper and mix well
4. Add your canned tomatoes alongside coconut milk and mix
5. Add chicken and give it a nice stir
6. Close up the lid then cook on **HIGH** pressure for about 8 minutes
7. Once done, pour coconut cream, tomato paste, and Garam Masala
8. Relish with some cilantro then serve with a sprinkle of sliced up almonds. Enjoy!

Chicken Korma

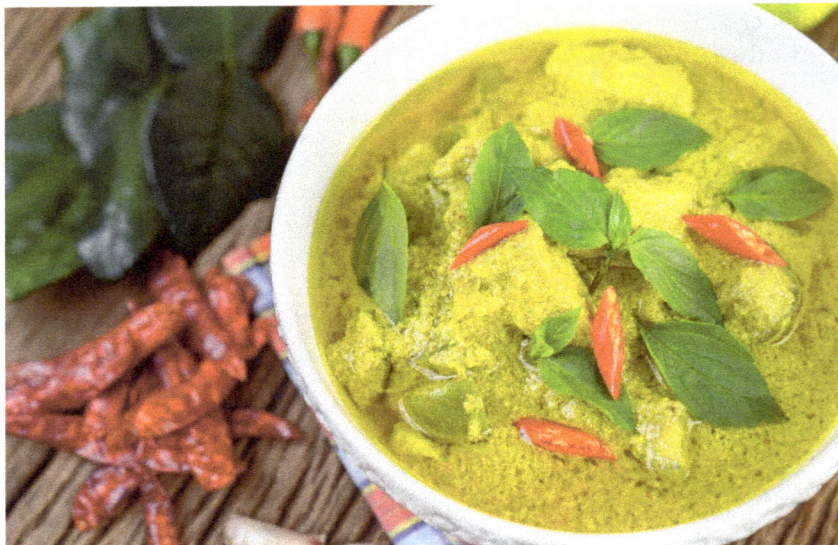

Preparation Time: 5 Minutes
Cooking Time: 10 Minutes
Servings: 6

Nutrition:
Calories:145,
Fat:4g,
Fiber:3g,
Carbs:11g,
Protein:4g
Ingredients:

- 1 pound of chicken
- For Sauce
- 1 ounce of cashews
- 1 small chopped onion
- ½ a cup of diced tomatoes
- ½ of green Serrano pepper
- 5 cloves of garlic
- 1 teaspoon of minced ginger
- 1 teaspoon of turmeric
- 1 teaspoon of Garam masala

- 1 teaspoon of cumin-coriander powder
- ½ a teaspoon of cayenne pepper
- ½ a cup of water

For topping

- 1 teaspoon of Garam masala
- ½ a cup of coconut milk
- ¼ cup of chopped cilantro

Directions:

1. Add the sauce fixings to a blender then blend them well
2. Pour the sauce to your Ninja Foodi. Place the chicken on top
3. Close up the lid then cook on HIGH pressure for 10 minutes
4. Release the pressure naturally. Take the chicken out and cut into bite-sized portions
5. Add coconut milk, Garam masala to the pot
6. Transfer the chicken back and garnish with cilantro. Enjoy!

Sauces, Dips and Dressings

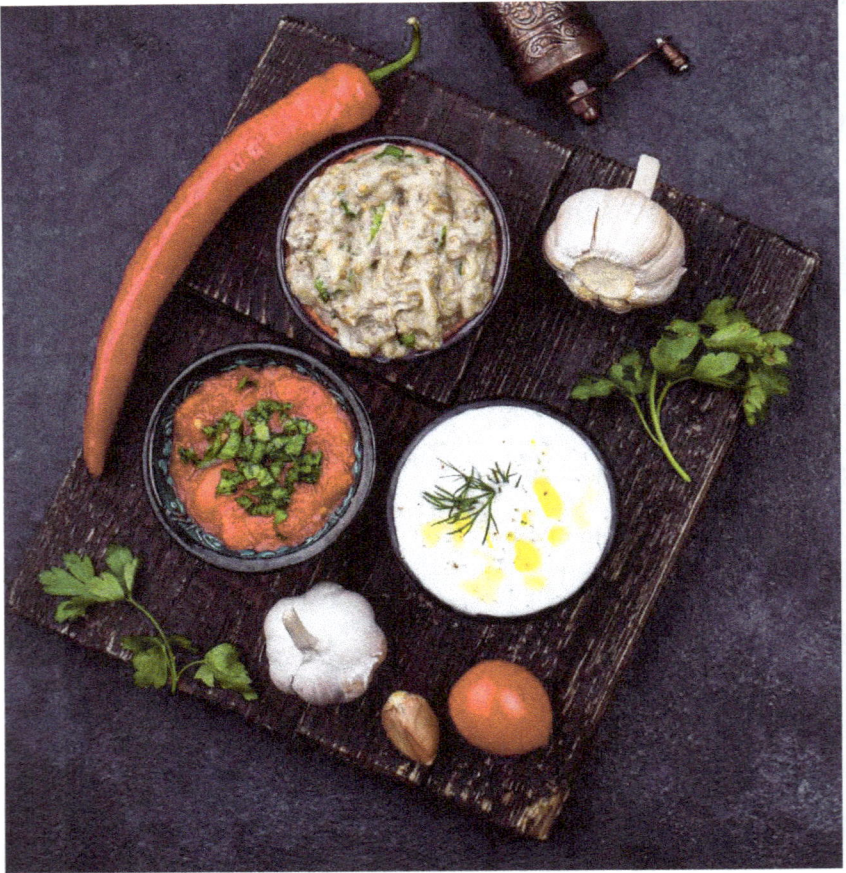

Hot Pepper Sauce

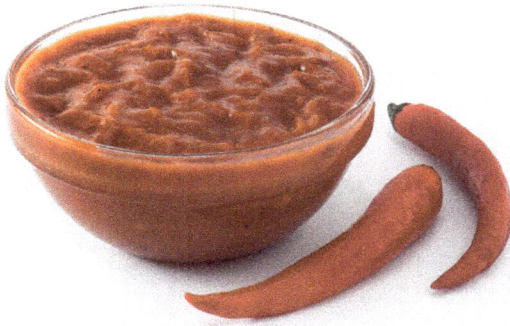

Preparation Time: 10 Minutes
Cooking Time: 20 Minutes
Servings: 8
Nutrition:
Calories: 20
Fat: 1.2g
Protein: 0.6g
Carbs: 4.4g
Fiber: 0.6g
Sodium: 12mg

Ingredients:

- 2 red hot fresh chiles, deseeded
- 2 dried chiles
- 2 garlic cloves, peeled
- ½ small yellow onion, roughly chopped
- 2 cups water
- 2 cups white vinegar

Directions:

1. Place all the fixings excluding the vinegar in a medium saucepan over medium heat. Allow to simmer for 20 minutes until softened.
2. Transfer the mixture to a food processor or blender. Stir in the vinegar and pulse until very smooth.
3. Serve immediately or transfer to a sealed container and refrigerate for up to 3 months.

Lemon-Tahini Sauce

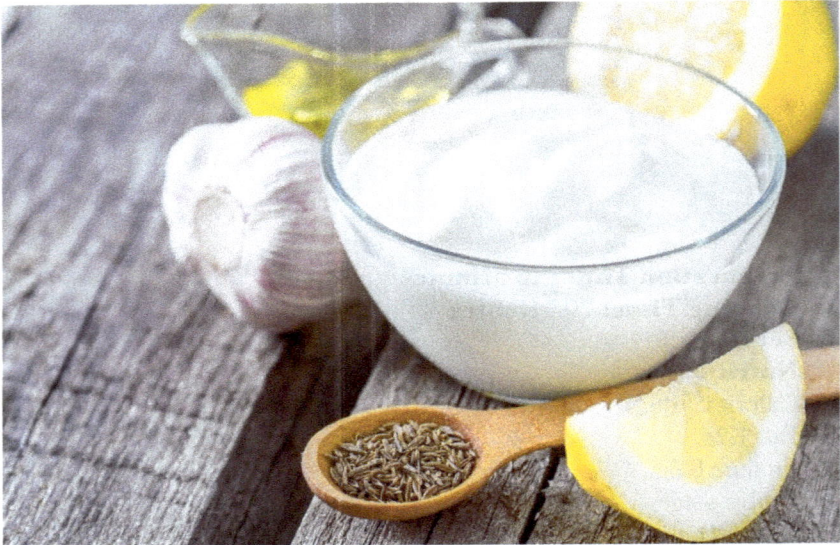

Preparation Time: 10 Minutes
Cooking Time: 0 Minutes
Servings: 4
Nutrition:
Calories: 179
Fat: 15.5g
Protein: 5.1g
Carbs: 6.8g
Fiber: 3.0g
Sodium: 324mg

Ingredients:

- ½ cup tahini
- 1 garlic clove, minced
- Juice and zest of 1 lemon
- ½ teaspoon salt, plus more as needed
- ½ cup warm water, plus more as needed

Directions:

1. Combine the tahini and garlic in a small bowl.
2. Add the lemon juice and zest and salt to the bowl and stir to mix well.
3. Fold in the warm water and whisk until well combined and creamy. Feel free to add more warm water if you like a thinner consistency.
4. Taste and add additional salt as needed.
5. Stock the sauce in a sealed container in the fridge for up to 5 days.

Peri-Peri Sauce

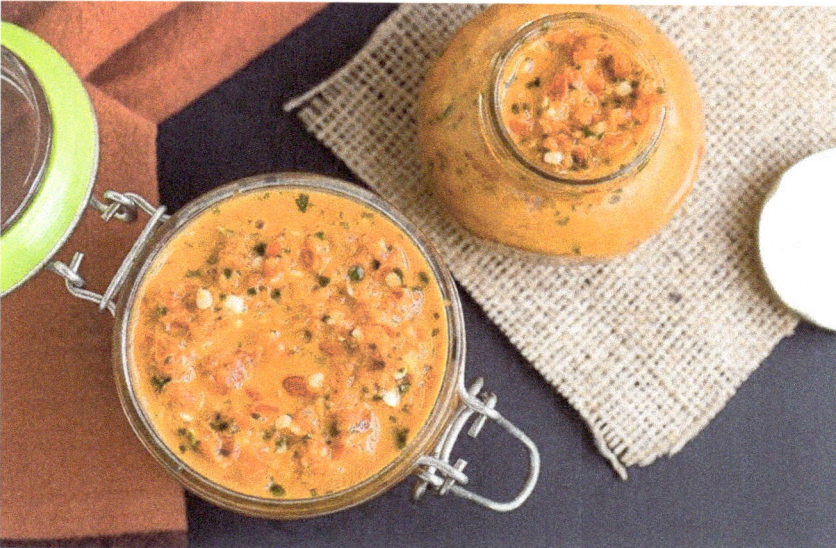

Preparation Time: 10 Minutes
Cooking Time: 5 Minutes
Servings: 4

Nutrition:

Calories: 98
Fat: 6.5g
Protein: 1.0g
Carbs: 7.8g
Fiber: 3.0g
Sodium: 295mg

Ingredients:

- 1 tomato, chopped
- 1 red onion, chopped
- 1 red bell pepper, deseeded and chopped
- 1 red chile, deseeded and chopped
- 4 garlic cloves, minced
- 2 tablespoons extra-virgin olive oil
- Juice of 1 lemon
- 1 tablespoon dried oregano
- 1 tablespoon smoked paprika
- 1 teaspoon sea salt

Directions:

1. Process all the fixings in a food processor or a blender until smooth.
2. Transfer the mixture to a small saucepan over medium-high heat and bring to a boil, stirring often.
3. Reduce the heat to medium and allow to simmer for 5 minutes until heated through.
4. You can store the sauce in an airtight container in the refrigerator for up to 5 days.

Peanut Sauce with Honey

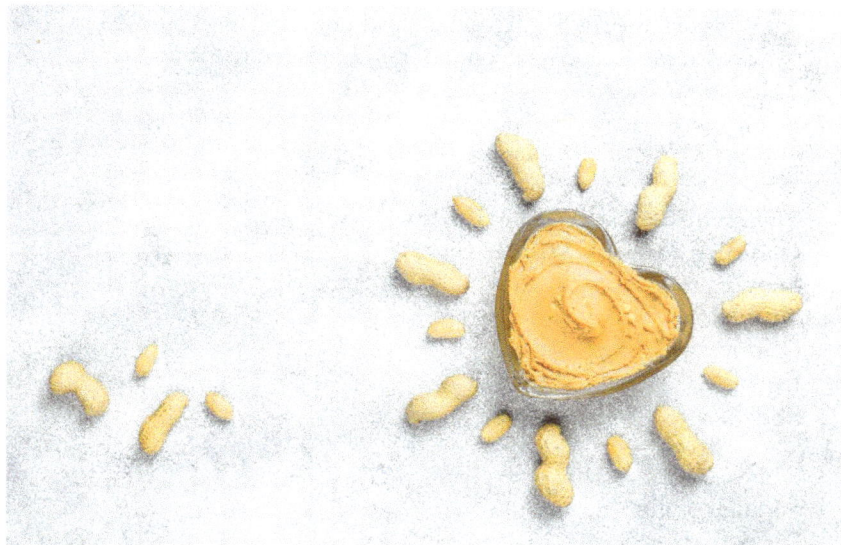

Preparation Time: 5 Minutes
Cooking Time: 0 Minutes
Servings: 4
Nutrition:
Calories: 117
Fat: 7.6g
Protein: 4.1g
Carbs: 8.8g
Fiber: 1.0g
Sodium: 136mg

Ingredients:

- ¼ cup peanut butter
- 1 tablespoon peeled and grated fresh ginger
- 1 tablespoon honey
- 1 tablespoon low-sodium soy sauce
- 1 garlic clove, minced
- Juice of 1 lime
- Pinch red pepper flakes

Directions:

1. Whisk all the fixings in a small bowl until well incorporated.
2. Transfer to an airtight container and refrigerate for up to 5 days.

Cilantro-Tomato Salsa

Preparation Time: 10 Minutes
Cooking Time: 0 Minutes
Servings: 6
Nutrition:
Calories: 17
Fat: 0g
Protein: 1.0g
Carbs: 3.9g
Fiber: 1.0g
Sodium: 83mg
Ingredients:

- 2 or 3 medium, ripe tomatoes, diced
- 1 serrano pepper, seeded and minced
- ½ red onion, minced
- ¼ cup minced fresh cilantro
- Juice of 1 lime
- ¼ teaspoon salt, plus more as needed

Directions:

1. Place the tomatoes, serrano pepper, onion, cilantro, lime juice, and salt in a small bowl and mix well.
2. Taste and add additional salt, if needed.
3. Store in a sealed vessel in the refrigerator for up to 3 days.

Simple Italian Dressing

Preparation Time: 5 Minutes
Cooking Time: 0 Minutes
Servings: 12
Nutrition:
Calories: 80
Fat: 8.6g
Protein: 0g

Carbs: 0g
Fiber: 0g
Sodium: 51m
Ingredients:

- ½ cup extra-virgin olive oil
- ¼ cup red wine vinegar
- 1 teaspoon dried Italian seasoning
- 1 teaspoon Dijon mustard
- ¼ teaspoon salt
- ¼ teaspoon freshly ground black pepper
- 1 garlic clove, minced

Directions:

1. Place all the fixings in a mason jar then cover. Shake vigorously for 1 minute until completely mixed.
2. Store in the refrigerator for up to 1 week.

Cheesy Pea Pesto

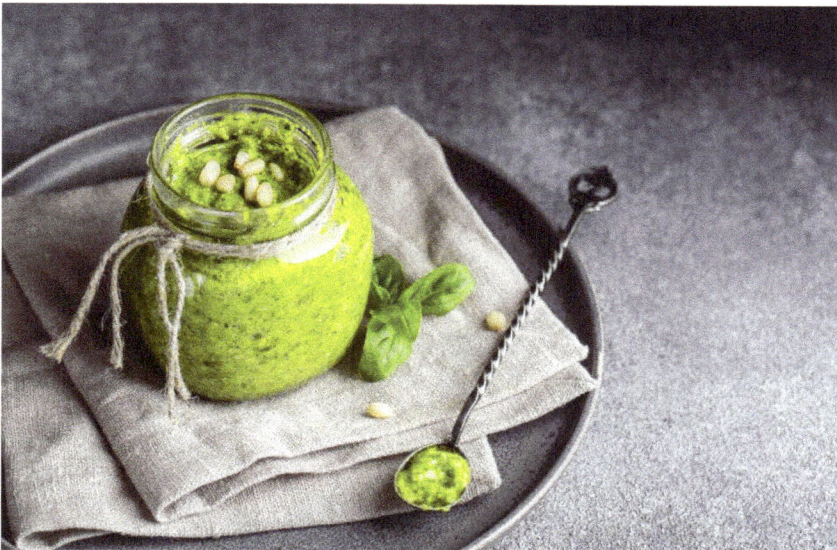

Preparation Time: 5 Minutes
Cooking Time: 0 Minutes
Servings: 4
Nutrition:
Calories: 247
Fat: 22.8g
Protein: 7.1g
Carbs: 4.8g
Fiber: 1.0g
Sodium: 337mg

Ingredients:

- ½ cup fresh green peas
- ½ cup grated Parmesan cheese
- ¼ cup extra-virgin olive oil
- ¼ cup pine nuts
- ¼ cup fresh basil leaves
- 2 garlic cloves, minced
- ¼ teaspoon sea salt

Directions:

1. Add all the fixings to a food processor or blender then pulse until the nuts are chopped finely.
2. Transfer to an airtight container and refrigerate for up to 2 days. You can also store it in ice cube trays in the freezer for up to 6 months.

Guacamole

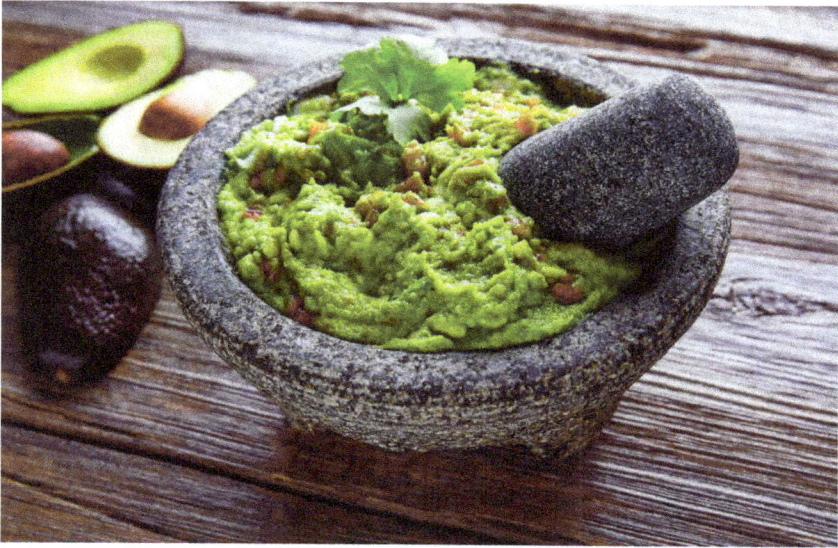

Preparation Time: 10 Minutes
Cooking Time: 0 Minutes
Servings: 6
Nutrition:
Calories: 81
Fat: 6.8g
Protein: 1.1g
Carbs: 5.7g
Fiber: 3.0g
Sodium: 83mg

Ingredients:

- 2 large avocados
- ¼ white onion, finely diced
- 1 small, firm tomato, finely diced
- ¼ cup finely chopped fresh cilantro
- 2 tablespoons freshly squeezed lime juice
- ¼ teaspoon salt
- Freshly ground black pepper, to taste

Directions:

1. Slice the avocados in half and take away the pits. Using a large spoon to scoop out the flesh and add to a medium bowl.
2. Mash the avocado flesh with the back of a fork, or until a uniform consistency is achieved. Add the onion, tomato, cilantro, lime juice, salt, and pepper to the bowl and stir to combine.
3. Serve instantly, or transfer to a sealed vessel and refrigerate until chilled.

Lentil-Tahini Dip

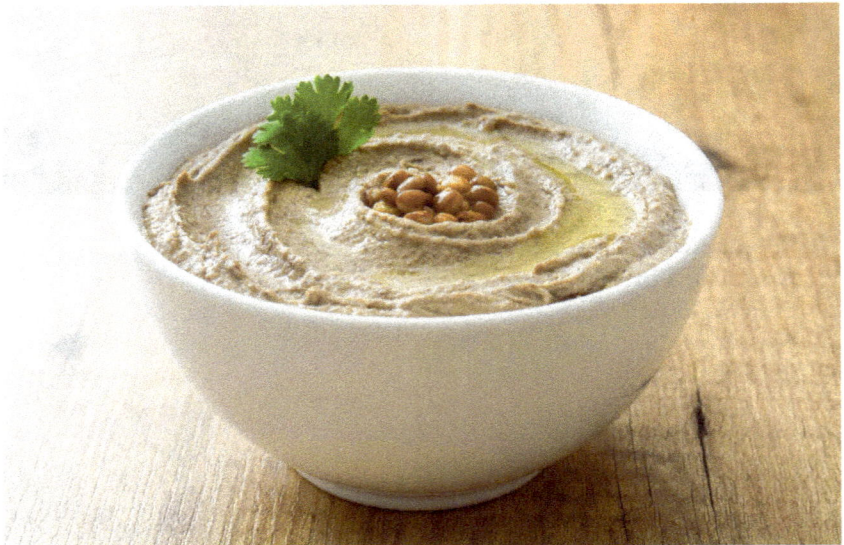

Preparation Time: 10 Minutes
Cooking Time: 15 Minutes
Servings: 8
Nutrition:
Calories: 100
Fat: 3.9g
Protein: 5.1g
Carbs: 10.7g
Fiber: 6.0g
Sodium: 106mg

Ingredients:

- 1 cup dried green or brown lentils, rinsed
- 2½ cups water, divided
- 1/3 cup tahini
- 1 garlic clove
- ½ teaspoon salt, plus more as needed

Directions:

1. Add the lentils in addition 2 cups of water to a medium saucepan and bring to a boil over high heat.
2. Once it twitches to boil, lessen the heat to low, and then cook for 14 minutes, stirring occasionally, or the lentils become tender but still hold their shape. You can drain any excess liquid.
3. Transfer the lentils to a food processor, along with the remaining water, tahini, garlic, and salt and process until smooth and creamy.
4. Taste and adjust the seasoning if needed. Serve immediately.

Lemon-Dill Cashew Dip

Preparation Time: 10 Minutes
Cooking Time: 0 Minutes
Servings: 4
Nutrition:
Calories: 37
Fat: 2.9g
Protein: 1.1g
Carbs: 1.9g
Fiber: 0g
Sodium: 36mg
Ingredients:

- ¾ cup cashews, saturated in water for at minimum 4 hours and drained well
- ¼ cup water
- Juice and zest of 1 lemon
- 2 tablespoons chopped fresh dill
- ¼ teaspoon salt, plus more as needed

Directions:

1. Put the cashews, water, lemon juice and zest in a blender and blend until smooth.
2. Add the dill and salt to the blender and blend again.
3. Taste and adjust the seasoning, if needed.
4. Transfer to an airtight container and refrigerate for at least 1 hour to blend the flavors.

Asian-Inspired Vinaigrette

Preparation Time: 5 Minutes
Cooking Time: 0 Minutes
Servings: 2
Nutrition:
Calories: 251
Fat: 26.8g
Protein: 0g
Carbs: 1.8g
Fiber: 0.7g
Sodium: 3mg
Ingredients:

- ¼ cup extra-virgin olive oil
- 3 tablespoons apple cider vinegar
- 1 garlic clove, minced
- 1 tablespoon peeled and grated fresh ginger
- 1 tablespoon chopped fresh cilantro
- 1 tablespoon freshly squeezed lime juice
- ½ teaspoon sriracha

Directions:

1. Add all the fixings in a small bowl then stir to mix well.
2. Serve immediately, or store covered in the refrigerator and shake before using.

Creamy Cucumber Dip

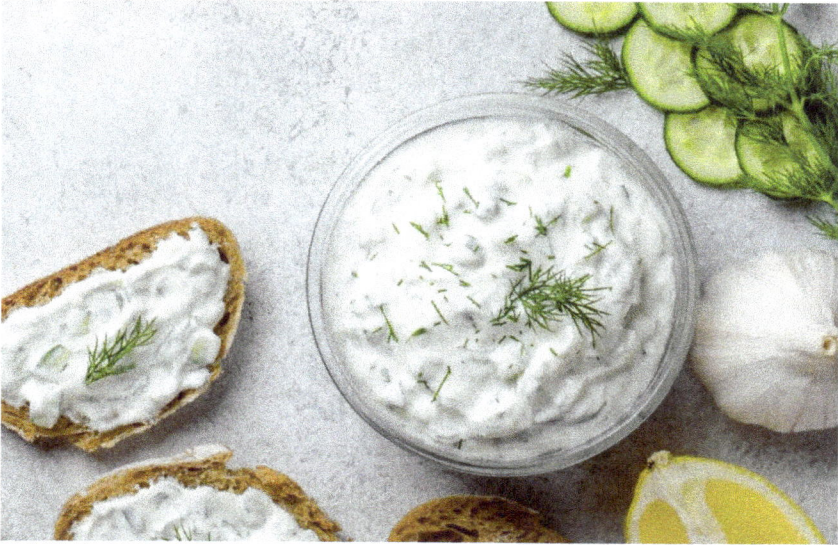

Preparation Time: 10 Minutes
Cooking Time: 0 Minutes
Servings: 6
Nutrition:
Calories: 47
Fat: 2.8g
Protein: 4.2g
Carbs: 2.7g
Fiber: 0g
Sodium: 103mg

Ingredients:

- 1 medium cucumber, peeled and grated
- ¼ teaspoon salt
- 1 cup plain Greek yogurt
- 2 garlic cloves, minced
- 1 tablespoon extra-virgin olive oil
- 1 tablespoon freshly squeezed lemon juice
- ¼ teaspoon freshly ground black pepper

Directions:

1. Put the grated cucumber in a colander set over a bowl and season with salt. Allow the cucumber to stand for 10 minutes. Using your hands, squeeze out as much liquid from the cucumber as possible. Transfer the grated cucumber to a medium bowl.
2. Add the yogurt, garlic, olive oil, lemon juice, and pepper to the bowl and stir until well blended.
3. Conceal the bowl with plastic wrap and refrigerate for at least 2 hours to blend the flavors.
4. Serve chilled.

Ranch-Style Cauliflower Dressing

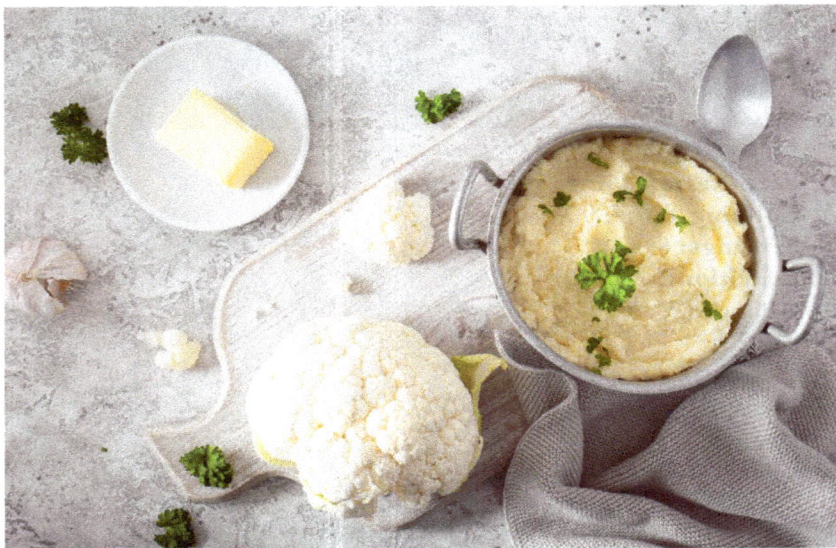

Preparation Time: 10 Minutes
Cooking Time: 0 Minutes
Servings: 8
Nutrition:
Calories: 41
Fat: 3.6g
Protein: 1.0g
Carbs: 1.9g
Fiber: 1.1g
Sodium: 148mg
Ingredients:

- 2 cups frozen cauliflower, thawed
- ½ cup unsweetened plain almond milk
- 2 tablespoons apple cider vinegar
- 2 tablespoons extra-virgin olive oil
- 1 garlic clove, peeled
- 2 teaspoons finely chopped fresh parsley
- 2 teaspoons finely chopped scallions (both white and green parts)
- 1 teaspoon finely chopped fresh dill
- ½ teaspoon onion powder
- ½ teaspoon Dijon mustard
- ½ teaspoon salt
- ¼ teaspoon freshly ground black pepper

Directions:

1. Place all the fixings in a blender then pulse until creamy and smooth.
2. Serve instantly, or handover to an airtight container to refrigerate for up to 3 days.

Parsley Vinaigrette

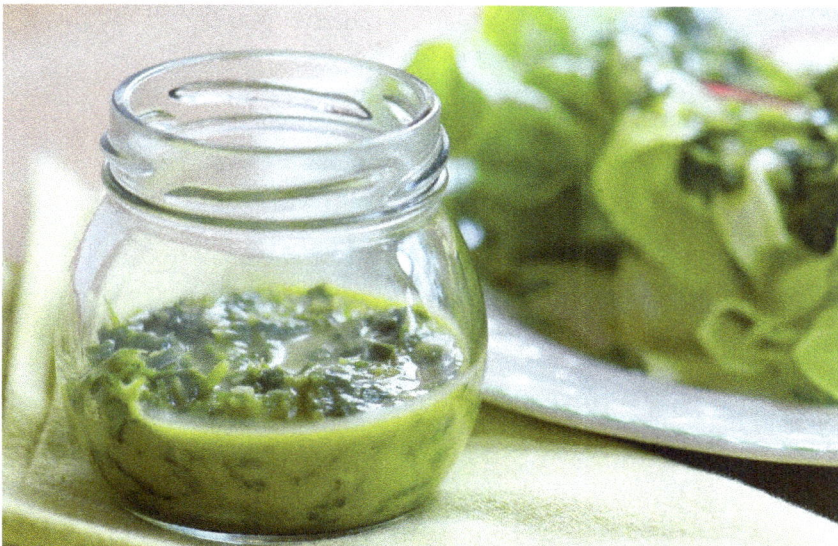

Preparation Time: 5 Minutes
Cooking Time: 0 Minutes
Servings: 2
Nutrition:
Calories: 92
Fat: 10.9g
Protein: 0g
Carbs: 0g
Fiber: 0g
Sodium: 75mg

Ingredients:

- ½ cup lightly packed fresh parsley, finely chopped
- 1/3 cup extra-virgin olive oil
- 3 tablespoons red wine vinegar
- 1 garlic clove, minced
- ¼ teaspoon salt, plus additional as needed

Directions:

1. Place all the fixings in a mason jar then cover. Shake vigorously for 1 minute until completely mixed.
2. Taste and add additional salt as needed.
3. Serve immediately or serve chilled.

Homemade Blackened Seasoning

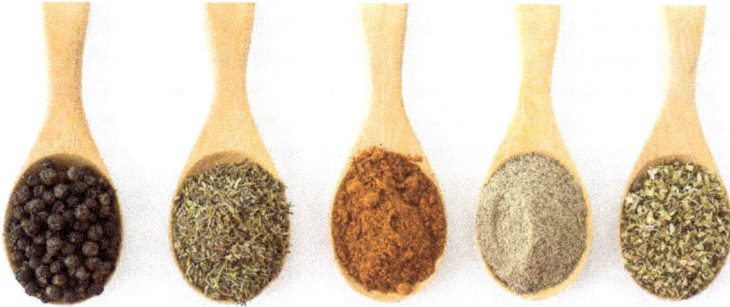

Preparation Time: 10 Minutes
Cooking Time: 0 Minutes
Servings: 2
Nutrition:
Calories: 22
Fat: 0.9g
Protein: 1.0g
Carbs: 4.7g
Fiber: 1.0g
Sodium: 2mg

Ingredients:

- 2 tablespoons smoked paprika
- 2 tablespoons garlic powder
- 2 tablespoons onion powder
- 1 tablespoon sweet paprika
- 1 teaspoon dried dill
- 1 teaspoon freshly ground black pepper
- ½ teaspoon ground mustard
- ¼ teaspoon celery seeds

Directions:

1. Add all the fixings to a small bowl then mix well.
2. Serve instantly, or handover to an airtight container and store in a cool, dry and dark place for up to 3 months.

Not Old Bay Seasoning

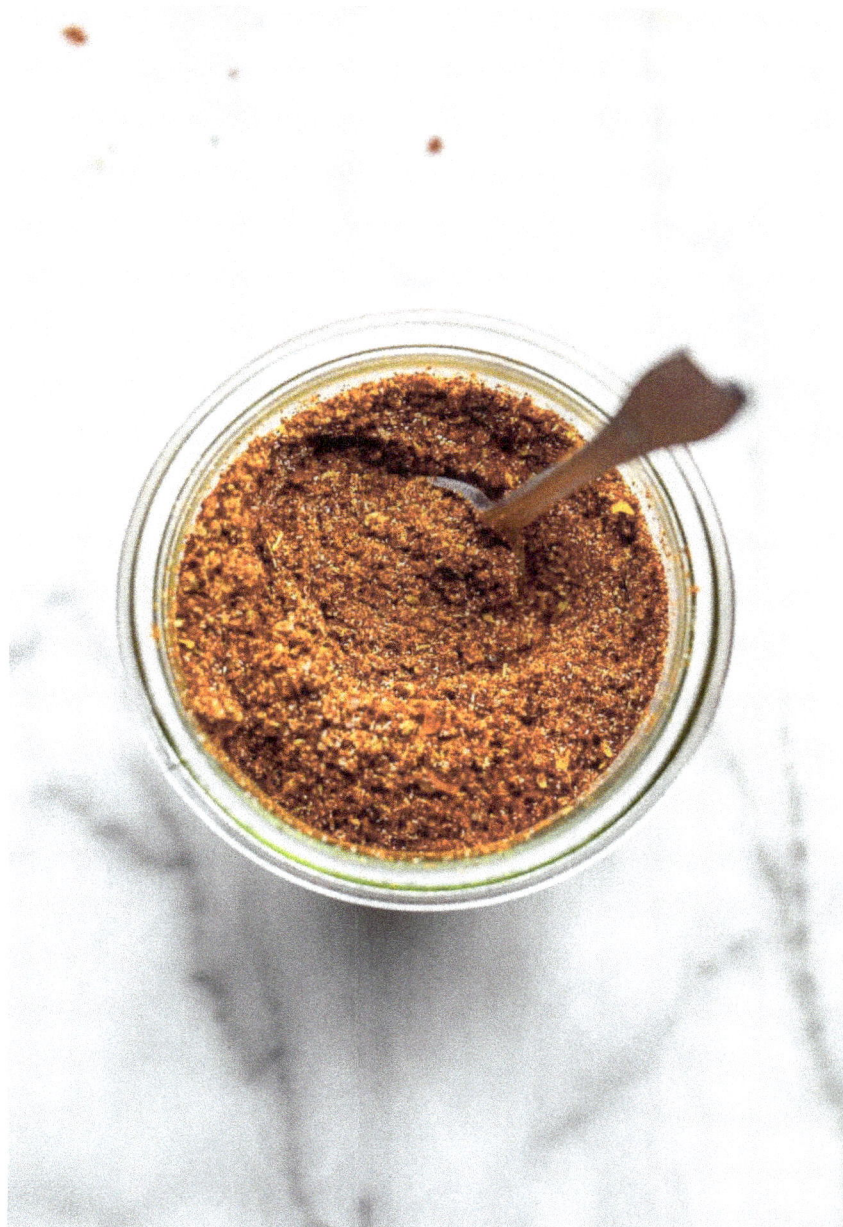

Preparation Time: 10 Minutes
Cooking Time: 0 Minutes
Servings: 2

Nutrition:
Calories: 26
Fat: 1.9g
Protein: 1.1g
Carbs: 3.6g
Fiber: 2.1g
Sodium: 3mg

Ingredients:

- 3 tablespoons sweet paprika
- 1 tablespoon mustard seeds
- 2 tablespoons celery seeds
- 2 teaspoons freshly ground black pepper
- 1 ½ teaspoons cayenne pepper
- 1 teaspoon red pepper flakes
- ½ teaspoon ground ginger
- ½ teaspoon ground nutmeg
- ½ teaspoon ground cinnamon
- ¼ teaspoon ground cloves

Directions:

1. Mix together all the ingredients in an airtight container until well combined.
2. You can store it in a cool, dry, and dark place for up to 3 months.

Tzatziki

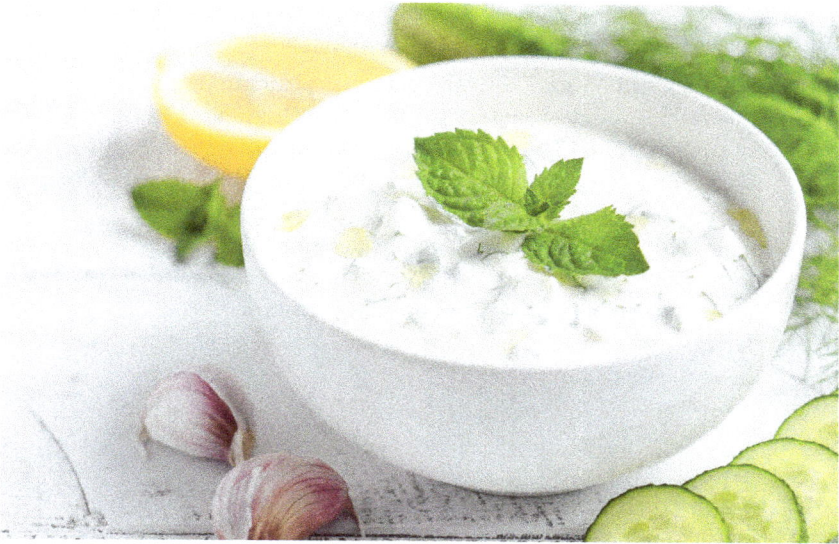

Preparation Time: 15 Minutes
Cooking Time: 0 Minutes
Servings: 6
Nutrition:
Calories: 286
Fat: 29.0g
Protein: 3.0g
Carbs: 5.0g
Fiber: 0g
Sodium: 615mg

Ingredients:

- ½ English cucumber, finely chopped
- 1 teaspoon salt, divided
- 1 cup plain Greek yogurt
- 8 tablespoons olive oil, divided
- 1 garlic clove, finely minced
- 1 to 2 tablespoons chopped fresh dill
- 1 teaspoon red wine vinegar
- ½ teaspoon freshly ground black pepper

Directions:

1. In a food processor, beat the cucumber until puréed. Place the cucumber on several layers of paper towels lining the bottom of a colander and sprinkle with ½ teaspoon of salt. Allow to drain for 10 to 15 minutes. Using your hands, squeeze out any remaining liquid.
2. In a medium bowl, whisk together the cucumber, yogurt, 6 tablespoons of olive oil, garlic, dill, vinegar, remaining ½ teaspoon of salt, and pepper until very smooth.
3. Drizzle with the residual 2 tablespoons of olive oil. Serve instantly or chill until ready to serve.

Pineapple Salsa

Preparation Time: 10 Minutes
Cooking Time: 0 Minutes
Servings: 6
Nutrition:
Calories: 55
Fat: 0.1g
Protein: 0.9g
Carbs: 12.7g
Fiber: 1.8g
Sodium: 20mg
Ingredients:

- 1 pound (454 g) fresh or thawed frozen pineapple, finely diced, juices reserved
- 1 white or red onion, finely diced
- 1 bunch cilantro or mint, leaves only, chopped
- 1 jalapeño, minced (optional)
- Salt, to taste

Directions:

1. Stir together the pineapple with its juice, onion, cilantro, and jalapeño (if desired) in a medium bowl. Season with salt to taste and serve.
2. The salsa can be refrigerated in an airtight container for up to 2 days.

Creamy Grapefruit and Tarragon Dressing

Preparation Time: 5 Minutes
Cooking Time: 0 Minutes
Servings: 6
Nutrition:
Calories: 86
Fat: 7.0g
Protein: 1.0g
Carbs: 6.0g
Fiber: 0g
Sodium: 390mg
Ingredients:

- ½ cup avocado oil mayonnaise
- 2 tablespoons Dijon mustard
- ½ teaspoon salt
- 1 teaspoon dried tarragon
- Zest and juice of ½ grapefruit
- ¼ teaspoon freshly ground black pepper
- 1 to 2 tablespoons water (optional)

Directions:

1. In a mason jar with lid, combine the mayonnaise, Dijon, tarragon, grapefruit zest and juice, salt, and pepper and whisk well with a fork until smooth and creamy. If a thinner dressing is preferred, thin out with water.
2. Serve instantly or chill until ready to serve.

Ginger Teriyaki Sauce

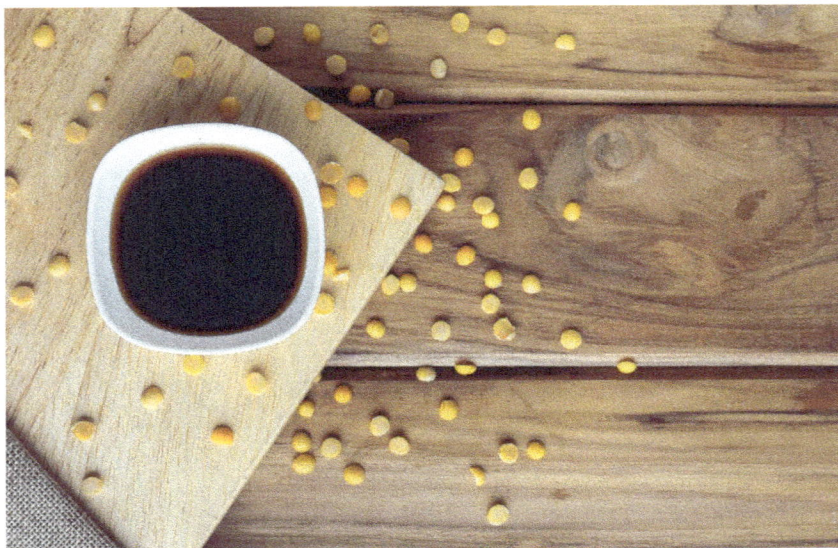

Preparation Time: 5 Minutes
Cooking Time: 0 Minutes
Servings: 2
Nutrition:
Calories: 37
Fat: 0.1g
Protein: 1.1g
Carbs: 12.0g
Fiber: 0g
Sodium: 881mg

Ingredients:

- ¼ cup pineapple juice
- ¼ cup low-sodium soy sauce
- 2 tablespoons packed coconut sugar
- 1 tablespoon grated fresh ginger
- 1 tablespoon arrowroot powder or cornstarch
- 1 teaspoon garlic powder

Directions:

1. Whisk the pineapple juice, soy sauce, coconut sugar, ginger, arrowroot powder, and garlic powder together in a small bowl.
2. Stock in a wrapped vessel in the fridge for up to 5 days.

Desserts

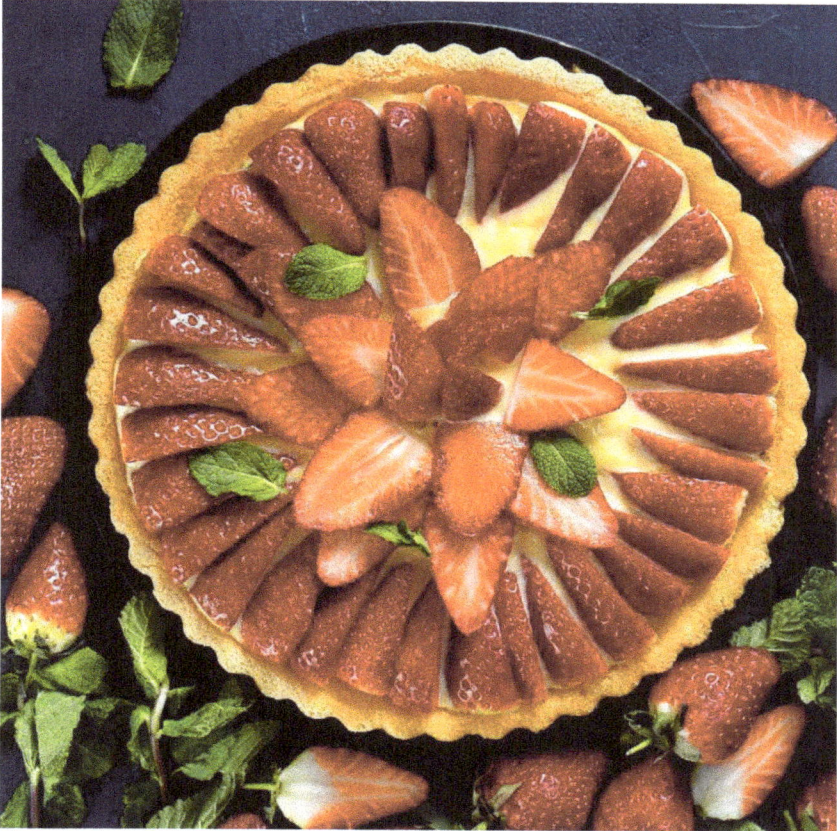

Stuffed Dried Figs

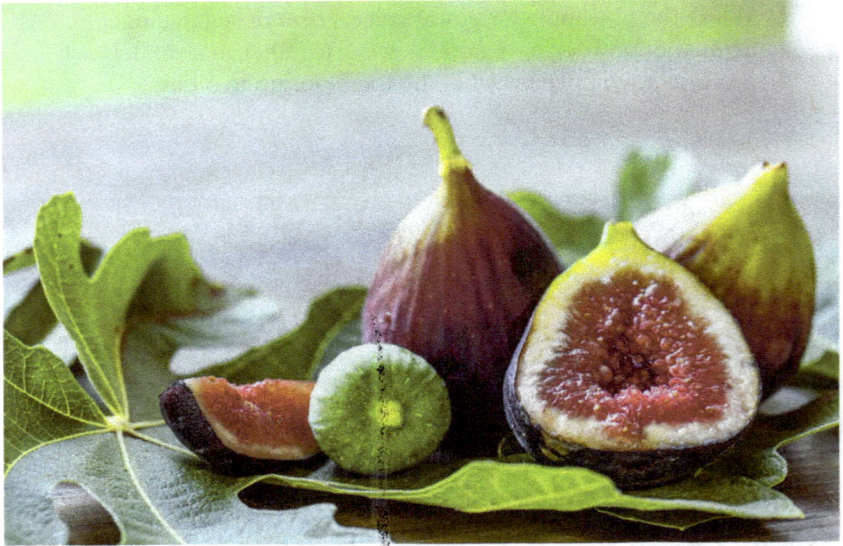

Preparation Time: 20 Minutes
Cooking Time: 0 Minutes
Servings: 4

Nutrition:
Calories: 110kcal
Carbs: 26
Fat: 3g,
Protein: 1g

Ingredients:

- 12 dried figs
- 2 Tbsps. thyme honey
- 2 Tbsps. sesame seeds
- 24 walnut halves

Directions:

1. Cut off the tough stalk ends of the figs.
2. Slice open each fig.

3. Stuff the fig openings with two walnut halves and close
4. Arrange the figs on a plate, drizzle with honey, and sprinkle the sesame seeds on it.
5. Serve.

Feta Cheesecake

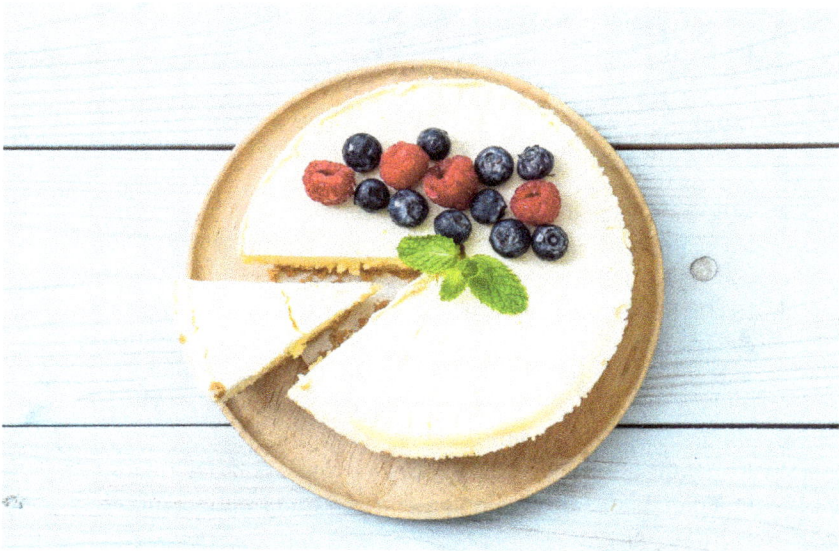

Preparation Time: 30 Minutes
Cooking Time: 90 Minutes
Servings: 12

Nutrition:
Calories: 98kcal
Carbs: 7g
Fat: 7g
Protein: 3g

Ingredients:

- 2 cups graham cracker crumbs (about 30 crackers)
- ½ tsp ground cinnamon

- 6 tbsps. unsalted butter, melted
- ½ cup sesame seeds, toasted
- 12 ounces cream cheese, softened
- 1 cup crumbled feta cheese
- 3 large eggs
- 1 cup of sugar
- 2 cups plain yogurt
- 2 tbsps. grated lemon zest
- 1 tsp vanilla

Directions:

1. Set the oven to 350°F.
2. Mix the cracker crumbs, butter, cinnamon, and sesame seeds with a fork. Move the combination to a springform pan and spread until it is even. Refrigerate.
3. In a separate bowl, mix the cream cheese and feta. With an electric mixer, beat both kinds of cheese together. Add the eggs one after the other, beating the mixture with each new addition. Add sugar, then keep beating until creamy. Mix in yogurt, vanilla, and lemon zest.
4. Bring out the refrigerated springform and spread the batter on it. Then place it in a baking pan. Pour water in the pan till it is halfway full.
5. Bake for about 50 minutes. Remove cheesecake and allow it to cool. Refrigerate for at least 4 hours.

Pear Croustade

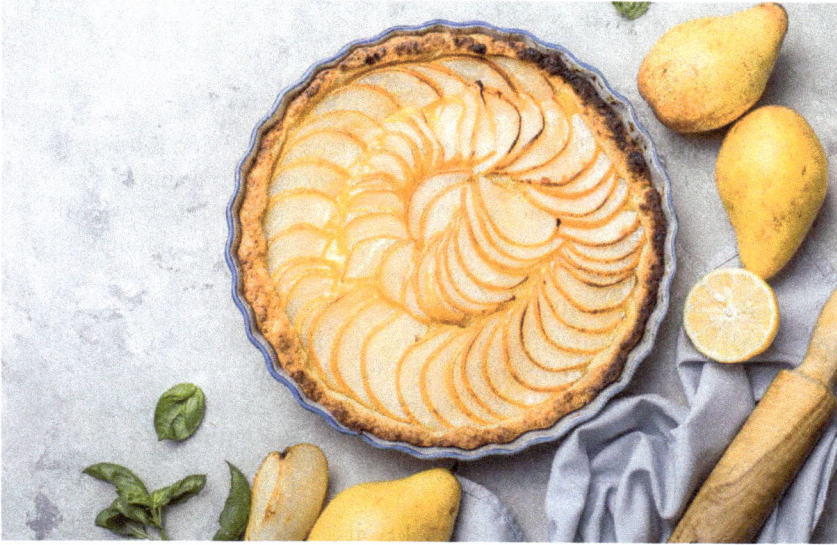

Preparation Time: 30 Minutes
Cooking Time: 60 Minutes
Servings: 10

Nutrition:
Calories: 498kcal
Carbs: 32g
Fat: 32g
Protein: 18g

Ingredients:

- 1 cup plus 1 tbsp. all-purpose flour, divided
- 4 ½ tbsps. sugar, divided
- 1/8 tsp salt
- 6 tbsps. unsalted butter, chilled, cut into ½ inch cubes
- 1 large-sized egg, separated
- 1 1/2 tbsps. ice-cold water
- 3 firm, ripe pears (Bosc), peeled, cored, sliced into ¼ inch slices
  1 tbsp. fresh lemon juice
- 1/3 tsp ground allspice

- 1 tsp anise seeds

Directions:

1. Pour 1 cup of flour, 1 ½ Tbsps. of sugar, butter, and salt into a food processor and combine the ingredients by pulsing.
2. Whisk the yolk of the egg and ice water in a separate bowl. Mix the egg mixture with the flour mixture. It will form a dough, wrap it, and set aside for an hour.
3. Set the oven to 400°F.
4. Mix the pear, sugar, leftover flour, allspice, anise seed, and lemon juice in a large bowl to make a filling.
5. Arrange the filling on the center of the dough.
6. Bake for about 40 minutes. Cool for about 15 minutes before serving.

Melomakarona

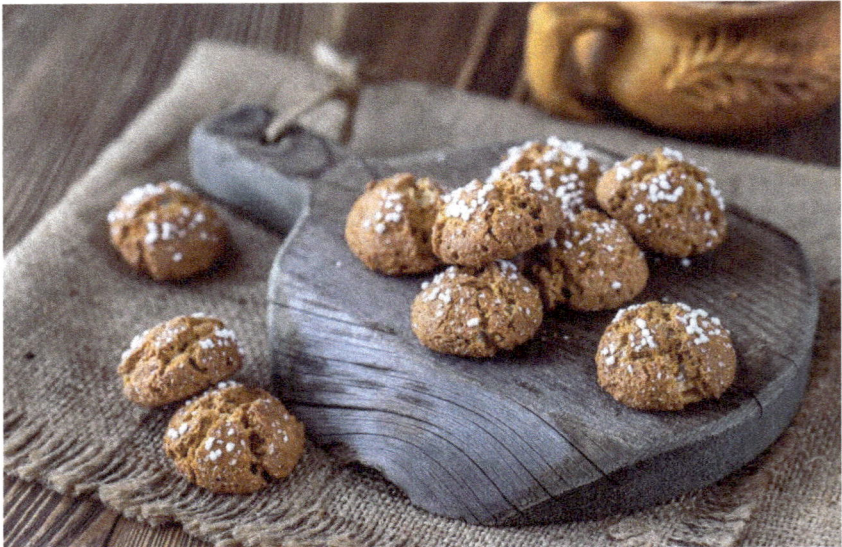

Preparation Time: 20 Minutes
Cooking Time: 45 Minutes
Servings: 20

Nutrition:

Calories: 294kcal
Carbs: 44g
Fat: 12g
Protein: 3g

Ingredients:

- 4 cups of sugar, divided
- 4 cups of water
- 1 cup plus 1 tbsp. honey, divided
- 1 (2-inch) strip orange peel, pith removed
- 1 cinnamon stick
- ½ cup extra-virgin olive oil
- ¼ cup unsalted butter,
- ¼ cup Metaxa brandy or any other brandy
- 1 tbsp. grated
- Orange zest
- ¾ cup of orange juice
- ¼ tsp baking soda
- 3 cups pastry flour
- ¾ cup fine semolina flour
- 1 ½ tsp baking powder
- 4 tsp ground cinnamon, divided
- 1 tsp ground cloves, divided
- 1 cup finely chopped walnut
- 1/3 cup brown sugar

Directions:

1. Mix 3 ½ cups of sugar, 1 cup honey, orange peel, cinnamon stick, and water in a pot and heat it for about 10 minutes.
2. Mix the sugar, oil, and butter for about minutes, then add the brandy, leftover honey, and zest. Then add a mixture of baking soda and orange juice. Mix thoroughly.
3. In a distinct bowl, blend the pastry flour, baking powder, semolina, 2 tsp of cinnamon, and ½ tsp. of cloves. Add the mixture to the mixer slowly. Run the mixer until the ingredients form a dough. Cover and set aside for 30 minutes.
4. Set the oven to 350°F

5. With your palms, form small oval balls from the dough. Make a total of forty balls.
6. Bake the cookie balls for 30 minutes, then drop them in the prepared syrup.
7. Create a mixture with the walnuts, leftover cinnamon, and cloves. Spread the mixture on the top of the baked cookies.

Loukoumades (Fried Honey Balls)

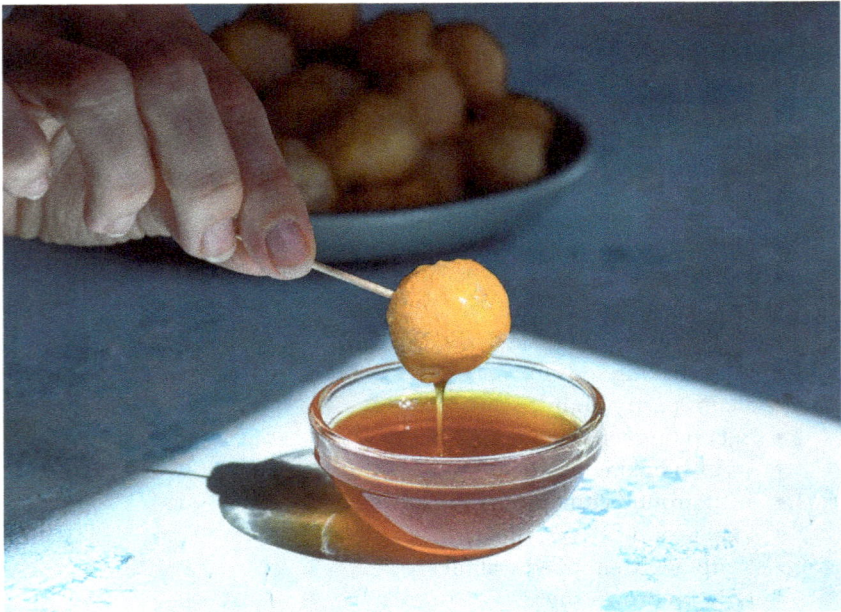

Preparation Time: 20 Minutes
Cooking Time: 45 Minutes
Servings: 10
Nutrition:
Calories: 355kcal
Carbs: 64g
Fat: 7g
Protein: 6g

Ingredients:

- 2 cups of sugar
- 1 cup of water
- 1 cup honey
- 1 ½ cups tepid water
- 1 tbsp. brown sugar
- ¼ cup of vegetable oil
- 1 tbsp. active dry yeast
- 1 ½ cups all-purpose flour, 1 cup cornstarch, ½ tsp salt
- Vegetable oil for frying
- 1 ½ cups chopped walnuts
- ¼ cup ground cinnamon

Directions:

1. Boil the sugar and water on medium heat. Add honey after 10 minutes. cool and set aside.
2. Mix the tepid water, oil, brown sugar,' and yeast in a large bowl. Allow it to sit for 10 minutes. In a distinct bowl, blend the flour, salt, and cornstarch. With your hands mix the yeast and the flour to make a wet dough. Cover and set aside for 2 hours.
3. Fry in oil at 350°F. Use your palm to measure the sizes of the dough as they are dropped in the frying pan. Fry each batch for about 3-4 minutes.
4. Immediately the loukoumades are done frying, drop them in the prepared syrup.
5. Serve with cinnamon and walnuts.

Crème Caramel

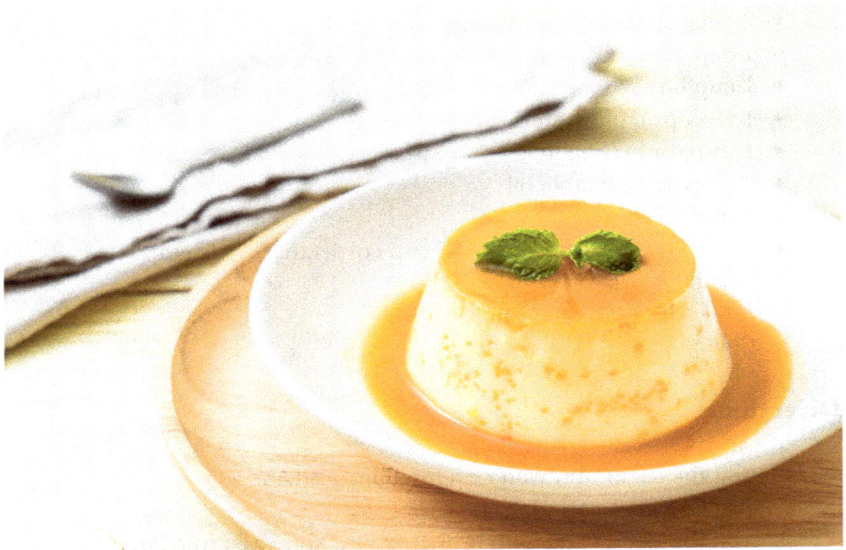

Preparation Time: 60 Minutes
Cooking Time: 60 Minutes
Servings: 12

Nutrition:
Calories: 110kcal
Carbs: 21g
Fat: 1g
Protein: 2g

Ingredients:

- 5 cups of whole milk
- 2 tsp vanilla extract
- 8 large egg yolks
- 4 large-sized eggs
- 2 cups sugar, divided
- ¼ cup 0f water

Directions:

1. Preheat the oven to 350°F
2. Heat the milk with medium heat wait for it to be scalded.
3. Mix 1 cup of sugar and eggs in a bowl and add it to the eggs.
4. With a nonstick pan on high heat, boil the water and remaining sugar. Do not stir, instead whirl the pan. When the sugar forms caramel, divide it into ramekins.
5. Divide the egg mixture into the ramekins and place in a baking pan. Increase water to the pan until it is half full. Bake for 30 minutes.
6. Remove the ramekins from the baking pan, cool, then refrigerate for at least 8 hours.

Galaktoboureko

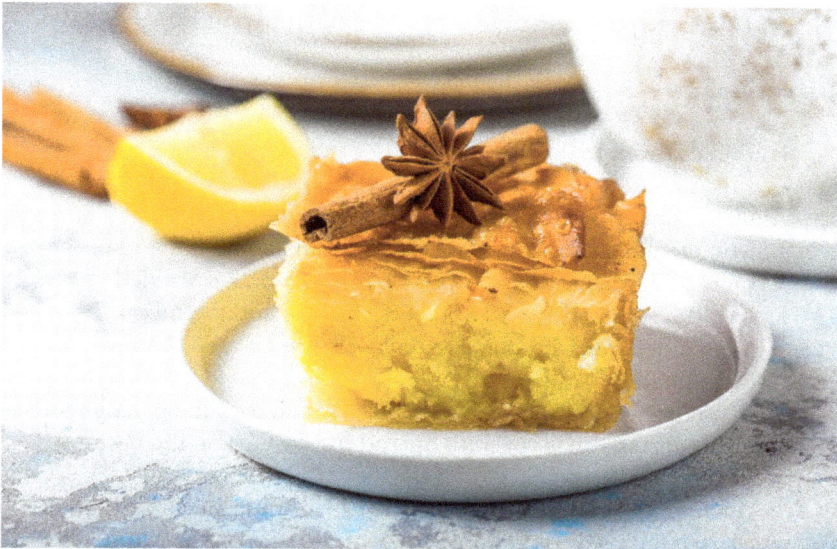

Preparation Time: 30 Minutes
Cooking Time: 90 Minutes
Servings: 12

Nutrition:
Calories: 393kcal
Carbs: 55g
Fat: 15g
Protein: 8g

. . .

Ingredients:

- 4 cups sugar, divided
- 1 tbsp. fresh lemon juice
- 1 cup of water
- 1 Tbsp. plus 1 ½ tsp grated lemon zest, divided into 10 cups
- Room temperature whole milk
- 1 cup plus 2 tbsps. unsalted butter, melted and divided into 2
- Tbsps. vanilla extract
- 7 large-sized eggs
- 1 cup of fine semolina
- 1 package phyllo, thawed and at room temperature

Directions:

1. Preheat oven to 350°F
2. Mix 2 cups of sugar, lemon juice, 1 ½ tsp of lemon zest, and water. Boil over medium heat. Set aside.
3. Mix the milk, 2 Tbsps. of butter, and vanilla in a pot and put-on medium heat. Remove from heat when milk is scalded
4. Mix the eggs and semolina in a bowl, then add the mixture to the scalded milk. Put the egg-milk mixture on medium heat. Stir until it forms a custard-like material.
5. Brush butter on each sheet then arrange all over the baking pan until everywhere is covered. Spread the custard on the bottom pile phyllo
6. Arrange the buttered phyllo all over the top of the custard until every inch is covered.
7. Bake for about 40 minutes. cover the top of the pie with all the prepared syrup. Serve.

Kourabiedes Almond Cookies

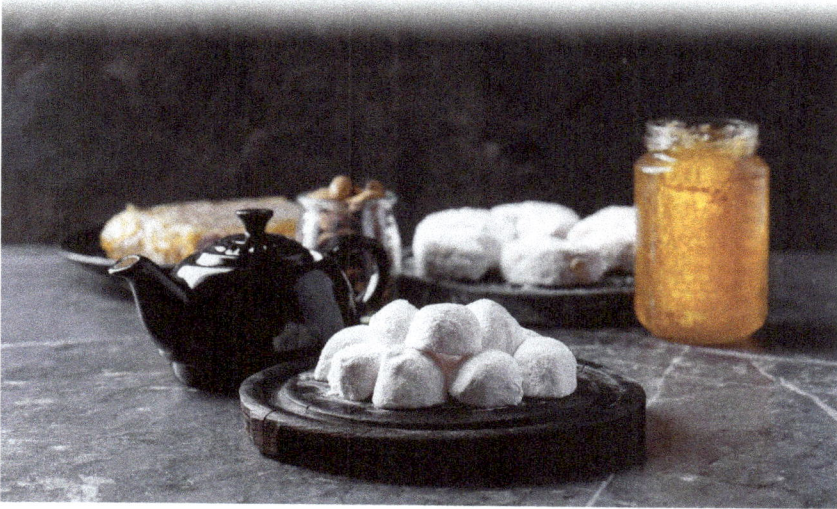

Preparation Time: 20 Minutes
Cooking Time: 50 Minutes
Servings: 20

Nutrition:
Calories: 102kcal
Carbs: 10g
Fat: 7g
Protein: 2g

Ingredients:

- 1 ½ cups unsalted butter, clarified, at room temperature 2 cups
- Confectioners' sugar, divided
- 1 large egg yolk
- 2 tbsps. brandy
- 1 1/2 tsp baking powder
- 1 tsp vanilla extract
- 5 cups all-purpose flour, sifted
- 1 cup roasted almonds, chopped

Directions:

1. Preheat the oven to 350°F
2. Thoroughly mix butter and ½ cup of sugar in a bowl. Add in the egg after a while. Create a brandy mixture by mixing the brandy and baking powder. Add the mixture to the egg, add vanilla, then keep beating until the ingredients are properly blended
3. Add flour and almonds to make a dough.
4. Roll the dough to form crescent shapes. You should be able to get about 40 pieces. Place the pieces on a baking sheet, then bake in the oven for 25 minutes.
5. Allow the cookies to cool, then coat them with the remaining confectioner's sugar.

Ekmek Kataifi

Preparation Time: 30 Minutes
Cooking Time: 45 Minutes
Servings: 10
Nutrition:
Calories: 649kcal
Carbs: 37g
Fat: 52g
Protein: 11g
Ingredients:

- 1 cup of sugar
- 1 cup of water
- 2 (2-inch) strips lemon peel, pith removed
- 1 tbsp. fresh lemon juice
- ½ cup plus 1 tbsp. unsalted butter, melted
- ½lbs. frozen kataifi pastry, thawed, at room temperature
- 2 ½ cups whole milk
- ½ tsp. ground mastiha
- 2 large eggs
- ¼ cup fine semolina
- 1 tsp. of cornstarch
- ¼ cup of sugar
- ½ cup sweetened coconut flakes
- 1 cup whipping cream

- 1 tsp. vanilla extract
- 1 tsp. powdered milk
- 3 tbsps. of confectioners' sugar
- ½ cup chopped unsalted pistachios

Directions:

1. Set the oven to 350°F. Grease the baking pan with 1. Tbsp of butter.
2. Put a pot on medium heat, then add water, sugar, lemon juice, lemon peel. Leave to boil for about 10 minutes. Reserve.
3. Untangle the kataifi, coat with the leftover butter, then place in the baking pan.
4. Mix the milk and mastiha, then place it on medium heat. Remove from heat when the milk is scalded, then cool the mixture.
5. Mix the eggs, cornstarch, semolina, and sugar in a bowl, stir thoroughly, then whisk the cooled milk mixture into the bowl.
6. Transfer the egg and milk mixture to a pot and place on heat. Wait for it to thicken like custard, then add the coconut flakes and cover it with a plastic wrap. Cool.
7. Spread the cooled custard-like material over the kataifi. Place in the refrigerator for at least 8 hours.
8. Strategically remove the kataifi from the pan with a knife. Take it away in such a way that the mold faces up.
9. Whip a cup of cream, add 1 tsp. vanilla, 1tsp. powdered milk, and 3 tbsps. Of sugar. Spread the mixture all over the custard, wait for it to harden, then flip and add the leftover cream mixture to the kataifi side.

Revani Syrup Cake

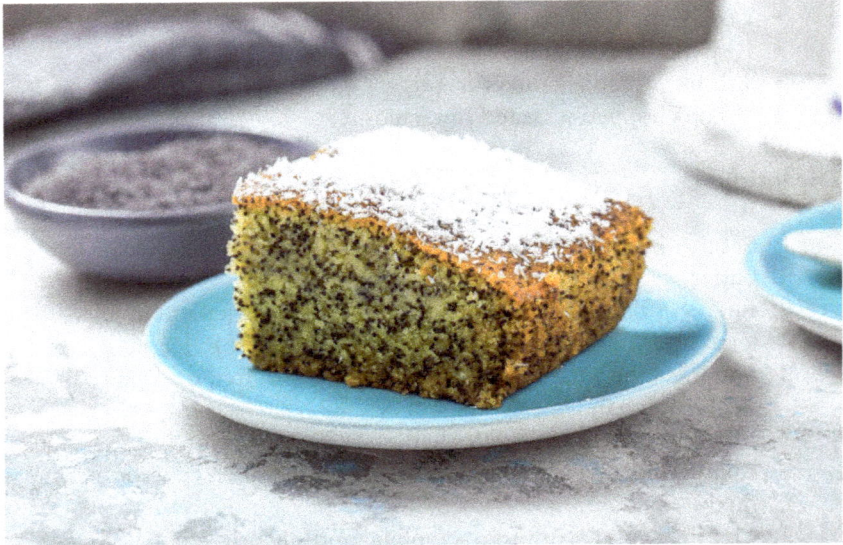

Preparation Time: 30 Minutes
Cooking Time: 3 Hours
Servings: 24

Nutrition:
Calories: 348kcal
Carbs: 55g
Fat: 9g
Protein: 5g

Ingredients:

- 1 tbsp. unsalted butter
- 2 tbsps. all-purpose flour
- 1 cup ground rusk or bread crumbs
- 1 cup fine semolina flour
- ¾ cup ground toasted almonds
- 3 tsp baking powder
- 16 large eggs
- 2 tbsps. vanilla extract
- 3 cups of sugar, divided

- 3 cups of water
- 5 (2-inch) strips lemon peel, pith removed
- 3 tbsps. fresh lemon juice
- 1 oz of brandy

Directions:

1. Preheat the oven to 350°F. Grease the baking pan with 1 Tbsp. of butter and flour.
2. Mix the rusk, almonds, semolina, baking powder in a bowl.
3. In another bowl, mix the eggs, 1 cup of sugar, vanilla, and whisk with an electric mixer for about 5 minutes. Add the semolina mixture to the eggs and stir.
4. Pour the stirred batter into the greased baking pan and place in the preheated oven.
5. With the remaining sugar, lemon peels, and water make the syrup by boiling the mixture on medium heat. Add the lemon juice after 6 minutes, then cook for 3 minutes. Remove the lemon peels and set the syrup aside.
6. After the cake is done in the oven, spread the syrup over the cake.
7. Cut the cake as you please and serve.

Almonds and Oats Pudding

Preparation Time: 10 Minutes
Cooking Time: 15 Minutes
Servings: 4
Nutrition:
Calories 174
Fat 12.1
Fiber 3.2
Carbs 3.9
Protein 4.8
Ingredients:

- 1 tablespoon lemon juice
- Zest of 1 lime
- 1 and ½ cups of almond milk
- 1 teaspoon almond extract
- ½ cup oats

- 2 tablespoons stevia
- ½ cup silver almonds, chopped

Directions:

1. In a pan, blend the almond milk plus the lime zest and the other ingredients, whisk, bring to a simmer and cook over medium heat for 15 minutes.
2. Split the mix into bowls then serve cold.

Chocolate Cups

Preparation Time: 2 Hours
Cooking Time: 0 Minutes
Servings: 6
Nutrition:
Calories 174
Fat 9.1
Fiber 2.2
Carbs 3.9
Protein 2.8
Ingredients:

- ½ cup avocado oil
- 1 cup, chocolate, melted
- 1 teaspoon matcha powder
- 3 tablespoons stevia

Directions:

1. In a bowl, mix the chocolate with the oil and the rest of the ingredients.
2. Whisk well and divide into cups.
3. Keep in the freezer for 2 hours before serving.

Mango Bowls

Preparation Time: 30 Minutes
Cooking Time: 0 Minutes

Servings: 4
Nutrition:
Calories 122
Fat 4
Fiber 5.3
Carbs 6.6
Protein 4.5
Ingredients:

- 3 cups mango, cut into medium chunks
- ½ cup of coconut water
- ¼ cup stevia
- 1 teaspoon vanilla extract

Directions:

1. In a blender, blend the mango plus the rest of the ingredients, pulse well.
2. Divide into bowls and serve cold.

Cocoa and Pears Cream

Preparation Time: 10 Minutes
Cooking Time: 0 Minutes
Servings: 4
Nutrition:
Calories 172
Fat 5.6
Fiber 3.5
Carbs 7.6
Protein 4
Ingredients:

- 2 cups heavy creamy
- 1/3 cup stevia
- ¾ cup cocoa powder
- 6 ounces dark chocolate, chopped
- Zest of 1 lemon

- 2 pears, chopped

Directions:

1. In a blender, blend the cream plus the stevia and the rest of the ingredients.
2. Blend well.
3. Divide into cups and serve cold.

Pineapple Pudding

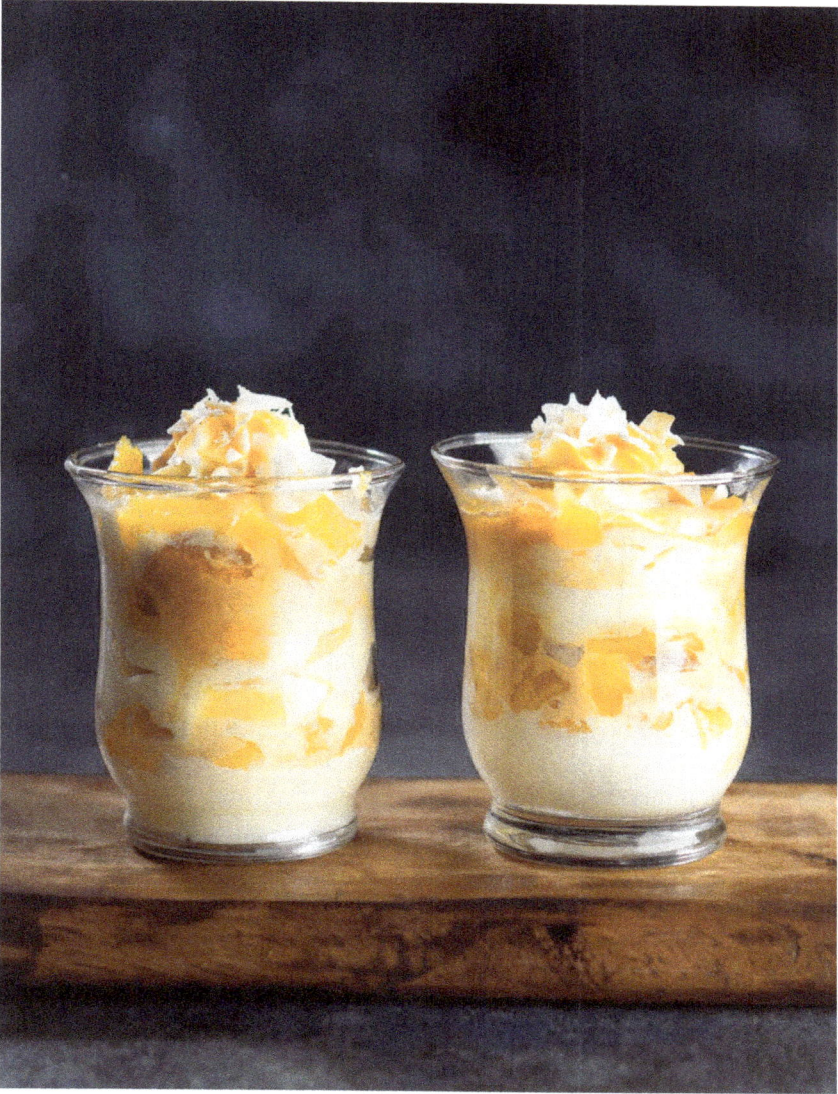

Preparation Time: 10 Minutes
Cooking Time: 40 Minutes
Servings: 4

Nutrition:
Calories 223

Fat 8.1
Fiber 3.4
Carbs 7.6
Protein 3.4

Ingredients:

- 3 cups almond flour
- ¼ cup olive oil
- 1 teaspoon vanilla extract
- 2 and ¼ cups stevia
- 3 eggs, whisked
- 1 and ¼ cup natural apple sauce
- 2 teaspoons baking powder
- 1 and ¼ cups of almond milk
- 2 cups pineapple, chopped
- Cooking spray

Directions:

1. In a bowl, blend the almond flour plus the oil and the rest of the ingredients except the cooking spray and stir well.
2. Grease a cake pan with the cooking spray, pour the pudding mix inside, introduce in the oven and bake at 370 degrees F for 40 minutes.
3. Serve the pudding cold.

Lime Vanilla Fudge

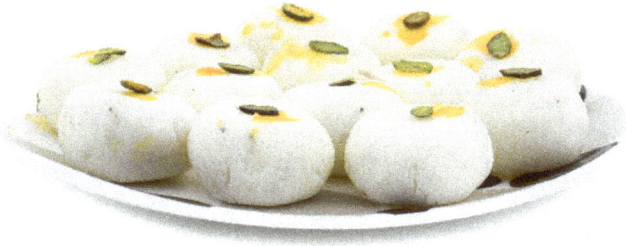

Preparation Time: 3 Hours
Cooking Time: 0 Minutes
Servings: 6

Nutrition:
Calories 200
Fat 4.5
Fiber 3.4
Carbs 13.5
Protein 5
Ingredients:

- 1/3 cup cashew butter
- 5 tablespoons lime juice
- ½ teaspoon lime zest, grated
- 1 tablespoons stevia

Directions:

1. In a bowl, mix the cashew butter with the other ingredients and whisk well.
2. Line a muffin tray with parchment paper, scoop 1 tablespoon

of lime fudge mix in each of the muffin tins and keep in the freezer for 3 hours before serving.

Blueberry Cake

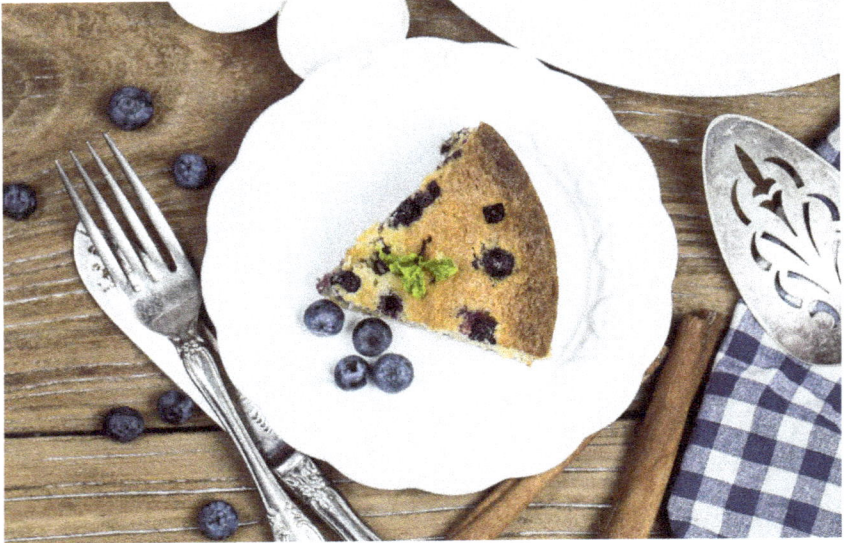

Preparation Time: 10 Minutes
Cooking Time: 30 Minutes
Servings: 6

Nutrition:
Calories 225
Fat 9
Fiber 4.5
Carbs 10.2
Protein 4.5
Ingredients:

- 2 cups almond flour
- 3 cups blueberries
- 1 cup walnuts, chopped
- 3 tablespoons stevia
- 1 teaspoon vanilla extract

- 2 eggs, whisked
- 2 tablespoons avocado oil
- 1 teaspoon baking powder
- Cooking spray

Directions:

1. In a bowl, blend the flour plus the blueberries, walnuts and the other ingredients except for the cooking spray, and stir well.
2. Grease a cake pan with the cooking spray, pour the cake mix inside, introduce everything in the oven at 350 degrees F and bake for 30 minutes.
3. Cool the cake down, slice and serve.

Orange and Apricots Cake

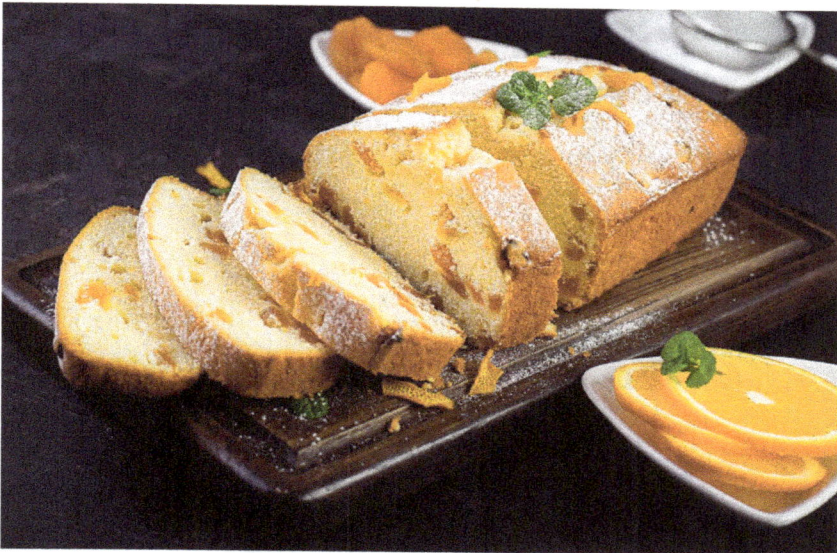

Preparation Time: 10 Minutes
Cooking Time: 20 Minutes
Servings: 8
Nutrition:
Calories 221
Fat 8.3
Fiber 3.4
Carbs 14.5

Protein 5

Ingredients:

- ¾ cup stevia
- 2 cups almond flour
- ¼ cup olive oil
- ½ cup almond milk
- 1 teaspoon baking powder
- 2 eggs
- ½ teaspoon vanilla extract
- Juice and zest of 2 oranges
- 2 cups apricots, chopped

Directions:

1. In a bowl, blend the stevia plus the flour and the rest of the ingredients, whisk and pour into a cake pan lined with parchment paper.
2. Introduce in the oven at 375 degrees F, bake for 20 minutes.
3. Cool down, slice and serve.

Almond Peaches Mix

Preparation Time: 10 Minutes
Cooking Time: 10 Minutes
Servings: 4
Nutrition:
Calories 135
Fat 4.1
Fiber 3.8
Carbs 4.1
Protein 2.3
Ingredients:

- 1/3 cup almonds, toasted
- 1/3 cup pistachios, toasted
- 1 teaspoon mint, chopped
- ½ cup of coconut water

- 1 teaspoon lemon zest, grated
- 4 peaches, halved
- 2 tablespoons stevia

Directions:

1. In a pan, combine the peaches with the stevia and the rest of the ingredients.
2. Simmer over medium heat for 10 minutes.
3. Divide into bowls and serve cold.

Mixed Berries Stew

Preparation Time: 10 Minutes
Cooking Time: 15 Minutes
Servings: 6
Nutrition:
Calories 172
Fat 7
Fiber 3.4
Carbs 8
Protein 2.3
Ingredients:

- Zest of 1 lemon, grated
- Juice of 1 lemon
- $\frac{1}{2}$ pint blueberries
- 1-pint strawberries halved
- 2 cups of water
- 2 tablespoons stevia

Directions:

1. In a pan, blend the berries plus the water, stevia and the other ingredients.
2. Bring to a simmer, cook over medium heat for 15 minutes.
3. Divide into bowls and serve cold.

Chicken Noodle Soup

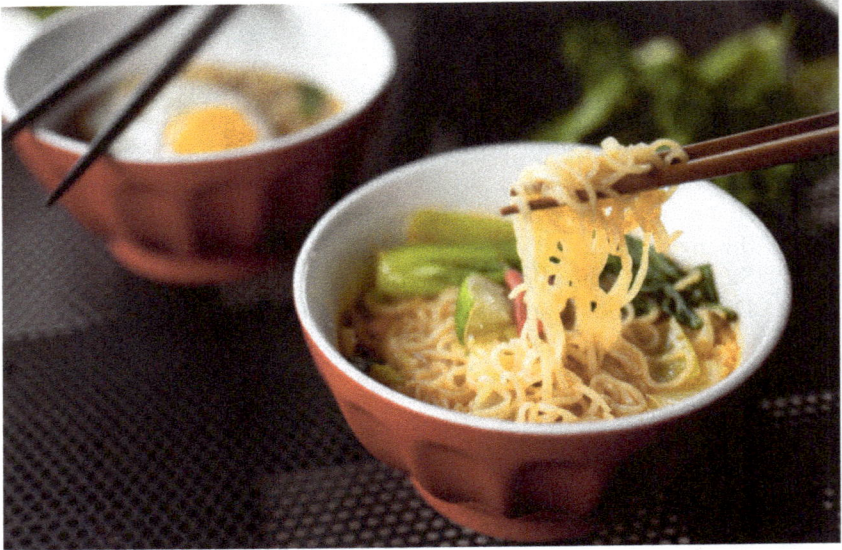

Who doesn't like chicken noodle soup on a cold winter's day, or even any other day when you feel like your immune system needs a boost of goodness? This recipe offers a light dinner option that is low in carbs and calories, a high-quality source of protein, and low mineral contents of sodium, potassium, and phosphorus. It also supports weight loss, diabetes, and is heart-healthy.

Time: 40 minutes

Serving Size: 10 servings (1 ¼ cups per serving)

Prep Time: 15 minutes

Cook Time: 25 minutes

Nutritional Info:

Calories: 185

Carbs: 14 g

Fat: 5 g

Protein: 21 g

Sodium: 361 mg

Potassium: 294 mg

Phosphorus: 161 mg

- 6 oz of noodles (uncooked)
- 8 cups of chicken broth (low-sodium)
- 4 cups of cooked chicken (cubed)
- 1 cup of carrots (diced)
- 1 cup of celery (diced)
- ½ cup of onion (diced)

- 3 tbsp of parsley (fresh)

Directions:

1. Bring the chicken broth to a boil in a large stockpot.
2. Add the diced vegetables, cubed chicken, and noodles to the pot.
3. Allow the soup ingredients to boil for at least 15 minutes until the noodles are properly cooked.
4. Garnish the soup with fresh parsley and serve it hot.

Food-prep tip: Store the chicken noodle soup in an airtight container in the refrigerator for up to 5 days, or freeze it for up to a month.

Vegetable Roast

This roast vegetable dish can be enjoyed on its own as a vegetarian meal, or with a lean source of protein like chicken breasts or white fish.

Time: 40 minutes

Serving Size: 6 servings (⅔ cup each)

Prep Time: 10 minutes

Cook Time: 30 minutes

Nutritional Info:

Calories: 141

Carbs: 14 g

Fat: 9 g

Protein: 2 g

Sodium: 7 mg

Potassium: 240 mg

Phosphorus: 48 mg

Ingredients:

- 2 cups of red potatoes (chopped into 1-inch cubes)
- ½ medium yellow bell pepper (diced)
- ½ medium red bell pepper (diced)
- 1 cup of button mushrooms (halved)
- ½ cup of zucchini (sliced)
- ¼ cup of olive oil
- 1 tbsp of garlic (minced)
- 2 tsp of rosemary (dried)
- 2 tsp of balsamic vinegar
- ½ tsp of black pepper

Directions:

1. Place the potatoes in a large pot of water on a stove over high

heat, to boil for at least 10 minutes. Once done, drain the water and cook the potatoes until they are tender.

2. Mix together all of the vegetable ingredients in a medium bowl, except for the potatoes.

3. Spread the vegetables out on a sheet pan and sprinkle them with black pepper. Allow them to roast for 15 minutes until the vegetables are slightly browned. Stir them a few times while cooking.

4. Add the potatoes and the vegetables to a large bowl and toss with the balsamic vinegar. Serve them hot.

Food-pep tip: Store the roasted vegetables in an airtight container in the refrigerator for up to 3 days. Add a source of high-quality protein, like chicken breasts or white fish, to build a complete meal.

Lettuce Wraps

For a heart-healthy and diet-friendly meal that is both satisfying and scrumptious to eat, these lettuce wraps are filled with good flavor — minus the carbs. Chicken breasts can be pre-cooked over the weekend and shredded in advance for this meal.

Time: 30 minutes
Serving Size: 4 (2 wraps each)
Prep Time: 15 minutes
Cook Time: 15 minutes
Nutritional Info:
Calories: 219
Carbs: 4 g
Fat: 15 g
Protein: 17 g
Sodium: 103 mg
Potassium: 225 mg
Phosphorus:130 mg
Ingredients:
- 8 oz of chicken breast (cooked, shredded)
- 8 large lettuce leaves
- 2 scallions (sliced)
- ¼ cup of red onion (diced)
- ¼ cup of button mushrooms (halved)
- ¼ cup of cilantro
- 2 tbsp of rice vinegar (unseasoned)
- 2 tbsp olive oil
- 1 tbsp sesame oil
- 2 tsp of soy sauce (low-sodium)

- 2 tsp of garlic (minced)

Directions:

1. Mix the shredded chicken in a bowl with the garlic. Toss the ingredients to combine well.
2. Sauté the mixture in a medium non-stick pan with scallions, garlic, sesame oil, olive oil, rice vinegar, and soy sauce. Cook over medium heat for 15 minutes, and stir the ingredients several times to prevent them from burning.
3. Remove the chicken and place it in a serving bowl. Place ¼ cup of chicken in each of the lettuce leaves. Add 1 to 2 tsp of onion, red bell pepper, mushrooms, cilantro, and parsley on top. Wrap the lettuce around the mixture and serve.

Food-prep tip: Store the lettuce cups in an airtight container in the refrigerator for up to 2 days. Alternatively, store the ingredients individually and arrange the lettuce cups when serving them.

Garlic Shrimp Pasta

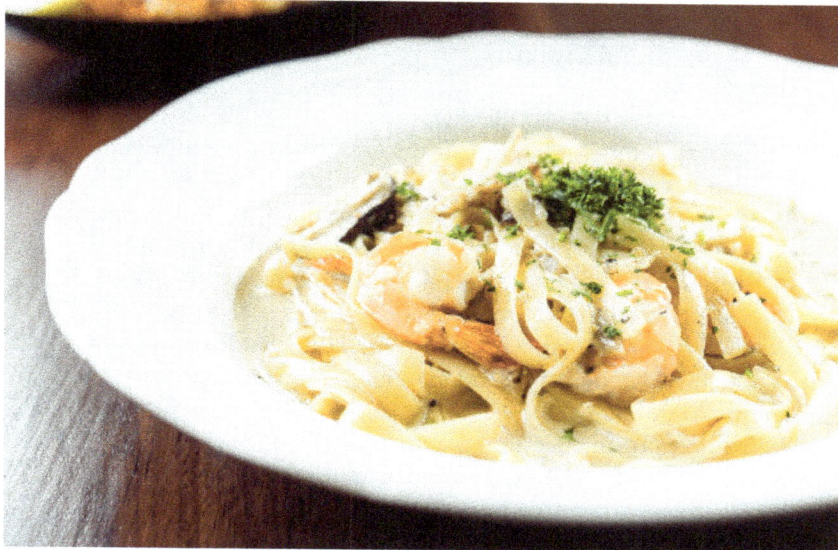

This pasta dish is delicious enough to leave you feeling like you've just had a cheat meal. However, the greatest thing of all is, you haven't. It's quick and easy to make and can serve an entire family.

Time: 20 minutes

Serving Size: 4 (1¼ cups each)

Prep Time: 5 minutes
Cook Time: 15 minutes
Nutritional Info:
Calories: 468
Carbs: 28 g
Fat: 28 g
Protein: 27 g
Sodium: 374 mg
Potassium: 469 mg
Phosphorus: 335 mg
Ingredients:
- 10 oz of cream cheese
- 4 oz of fettuccine (uncooked)
- ¾ oz of shrimp
- 1 ¾ cups of broccoli florets
- ¼ cup of red bell pepper (diced)
- ¼ cup of creamer
- ¼ cup of lemon juice
- 1 garlic clove (minced)
- ½ tsp of garlic powder
- ¾ tsp of black pepper

Directions:

1. Fill a medium pot three-quarters full with water and bring to a boil over high heat. Once the water is boiling, add the fettuccine pasta to the pot. Allow it to cook for 8 to 10 minutes, adding the broccoli for the final 3 minutes before removing it from the heat, draining the pasta, and setting it aside. Close the pot with a lid to lock in the heat.
2. Cook the shrimp and garlic over medium heat for 3 minutes in a non-stick pan, stirring often, until the shrimp is properly heated through.
3. Add the cream cheese, lemon juice, garlic powder, and black pepper. Cook the ingredients for 2 minutes.
4. Add the shrimp mixture to the pasta mixture, and stir to combine everything well.
5. Add a dash of black pepper to finish off the meal, and serve it hot.

Food-prep tip: Store the pasta dish in an airtight container in the refrigerator for up to 3 days.

Meat, Beans, and Corn Chili

This meat, beans, and corn chili is delectable, and surprisingly low in calories, too. It contains an excellent source of protein and is perfect if you are tight on time and looking to prepare a hot dish for a cold winter day. If this meal doesn't feel like comfort in a bowl, then what does! Additionally, it can be enjoyed with a nice crisp piece of ciabatta bread.

Time: 25 minutes
Serving Size: 8
Prep Time: 2 minutes
Cook Time: 23 minutes
Nutritional Info:
Calories: 217
Carbs: 18.7 g
Fat: 8.7 g
Protein: 17.5 g
Sodium: 268 mg
Potassium: 252 mg
Phosphorus: 168 mg
Ingredients:
- 15 oz of kidney beans
- 14.5 oz of roasted tomatoes (diced)
- 1 oz of beef (ground)
- 1 oz of turkey (ground)
- 2 cups of chicken stock
- 1 onion (diced)
- 3 tbsp tamari (gluten-free)
- 1 tbsp of avocado oil
- 1 tbsp of molasses
- 1 tbsp of kosher salt
- ½ tbsp of tomato paste
- 2 tsp of onion powder
- 2 cups of sweet corn (frozen)
- 1 ½ tsp of paprika
- 1 tsp of apple cider vinegar
- 1 tsp of cumin
- 1 tsp of garlic powder

Directions:

1. Heat the oil in a large stockpot over medium heat and cook the onion for around 5 minutes, until it is golden brown.
2. Add the ground beef and turkey and cook the meat until it is cooked through. Using the spatula, break everything into small pieces.

3. Add the kidney beans, roasted tomatoes, chicken stock, tamari, avocado oil, molasses, salt, tomato paste, onion powder, sweet corn, paprika, apple cider vinegar, cumin, and garlic powder to the pot's contents, and mix everything to combine well. Bring to a boil and reduce the heat for it to simmer. Cover the pot and let simmer for up to 15 minutes.
4. Switch off the heat, and add black pepper to serve.

Food-prep tip: Store the chili in an airtight glass container in the refrigerator for up to 5 days.

Chicken Veggie Stir-Fry

For an Asian-inspired stir-fry dish, prepare this once a week for two people to keep for up to 3 days. This dish is low in calories and offers a quick and easy dinner that you can make within 30 minutes.

Time: 25 minutes
Serving Size: 6
Prep Time: 5 minutes
Cook Time: 10 minutes
Nutritional Info:
Calories: 279
Carbs: 38 g
Fat: 6 g
Protein: 17 g
Sodium: 196 mg
Potassium: 349 mg
Phosphorus: 180 mg
Ingredients:
- 12 oz of chicken breast (boneless and skinless)
- 3 cups of mixed vegetables (frozen)
- 3 cups of rice (cooked)
- 3 tbsp of honey
- 3 tbsp of pineapple juice
- 3 tbsp of vinegar
- 2 tbsp of olive oil
- 1 ½ tbsp of soy sauce (low-sodium)
- 1 ½ tbsp of cornstarch

Directions:

1. Rinse the chicken breasts and pat them dry before cutting them into 1-inch pieces. Set aside for later.
2. For the sauce, combine the vinegar, pineapple juice, honey, cornstarch, and soy sauce. Set the sauce aside.

3. Pour the olive oil into a large non-stick pan, and add more oil to cook the frozen vegetables in the pan for 3 to 5 minutes. Remove the vegetables from the heat once they are crisp and tender.

4. Add the chicken to the hot non-stick pan and stir-fry it for 4 minutes, or until fully cooked. Remove the chicken from the center of the pan, and stir in the sauce set aside earlier. Cook and stir the pan contents until the sauce is thick and makes bubbles.

5. Add the cooked vegetables back to the pan, and the ingredients together until everything is well coated. Continue cooking, stirring the contents, for 1 more minute.

6. Serve the stir-fry over a portion of rice.

Food-prep tip: Store the stir-fry and rice in separate sealed, airtight containers in the refrigerator for up to 3 days. Heat it up for an easy dinner after a long day at work.

Coconut Bean Curry

This curry dinner is infused with incredible flavors and is quick and easy to make to serve two people.

Time: 15 minutes
Serving Size: 2
Prep Time: 5 minutes
Cook Time: 10 minutes
Nutrition Info:
Calories: 418
Carbs: 34.4 g
Fat: 29 g
Protein: 10.6 g
Sodium: 469 mg
Potassium: 600 mg
Phosphorus: 398 mg
Ingredients:
- 15 oz of crushed tomatoes (canned)
- 15 oz of kidney beans (canned, drained)
- 14 oz of coconut milk (canned)
- 2 garlic cloves (minced)
- 1 cup of brown rice (cooked)
- 1 white onion (diced)
- 2 tbsp of vegetable oil (30 ml)
- 2 tbsp of ginger (grated)
- 1 tbsp of masala

- 1 tsp of soy sauce
- 1 tsp of fresh cilantro
- ½ tsp of lime juice

Directions:

1. In a large pot, heat the oil over medium to high heat and add the onion, ginger, garlic, and masala to the pot. Cook until the onion softens, which should be 4 to 5 minutes.
2. Add crushed tomatoes, kidney beans, coconut milk, and soy sauce to the pot, and allow it to simmer. Cook the contents for 10 minutes for the flavors to blend properly. Taste-test the curry and add more salt to increase the flavors.
3. Heat up the brown rice, then top with curry, fresh cilantro, and a drizzle of lime juice.

Food-prep tip: Store the bean curry and rice in separate airtight containers in the refrigerator for up to 4 days.

Crusted Steak Pie

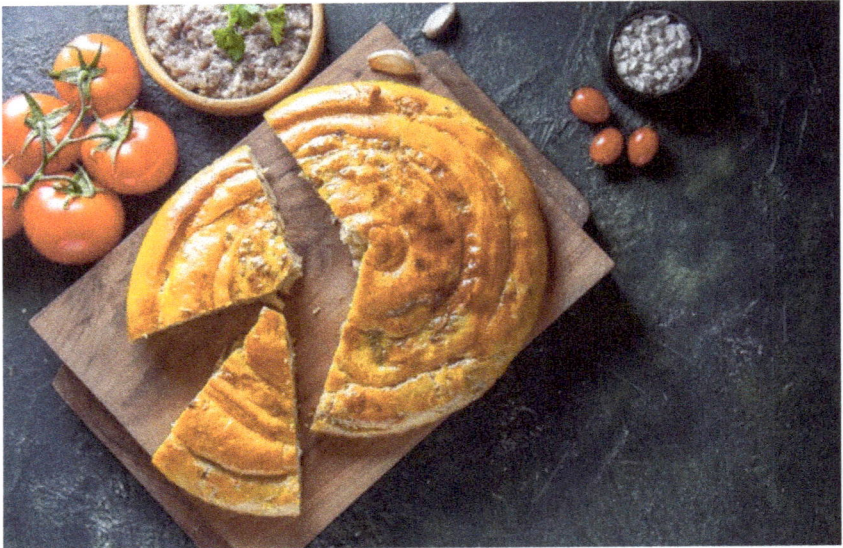

This pot pie is a classic and traditional meal that can be enjoyed among family on its own or with a side of roasted vegetables.

Time: 1 hour and 40 minutes
Serving Size: 6
Prep Time: 10 minutes

Cook Time: 90 minutes
Nutritional Info:
Calories: 488
Carbs: 50.6 g
Fat: 18.2 g
Protein: 9.9 g
Sodium: 345 mg
Potassium: 288 mg
Phosphorus: 195 mg
Ingredients:
- 9" pastry (for the pie's crust)
- 2 lbs of steak (cubed)
- 2 onions (diced)
- 1 bay leaf
- 4 cups of potatoes (diced)
- 2 cups of water
- 6 tbsp of flour (all-purpose)
- 2 tbsp of lard
- 2 tsp of Worcestershire sauce
- 2 tsp of kosher salt
- ½ tsp of thyme (dried)
- ¼ tsp of black pepper

Directions:

1. In a large stew pot, add in the steak with the lard, followed by the onion, bay leaf, Worcestershire sauce, kosher salt, thyme, and black pepper. Then, add 1 ½ cups of water, bring to a boil, and allow it to simmer for an hour until the meat and vegetables are tender.
2. Add in the potatoes, and continue to simmer the pot contents until the potatoes are tender, which should take about 30 minutes.
3. Combine the flour and the remaining ½ cup of water. Stir it into the mixture, and continue stirring and cooking until the mixture thickens. Once done, pour it into a large pie dish.
4. Roll out the pastry so that it is bigger than the size of the casserole dish, and place it over the mixture. Trim the dough that hangs over the dish and fold it to seal. Cut a few steam vents in the center of the pie.
5. Bake the steak pie at 425°F for up to 30 minutes or until it is lightly browned. Serve hot.

Food-prep tip: Store the pie in an airtight container in the refrigerator for up to 3 days.

Crispy Salsa Tacos

Prepare these Mexican-inspired salsa tacos for a spicy and tasty dinner. It is a gluten-free, vegan option.

Time: 30 minutes

Serving Size: 8

Prep Time: 10 minutes

Cook Time: 20 minutes

Nutritional Info:

Calories: 130

Carbs: 20 g

Fat: 4.6 g

Protein: 3.8 g

Sodium: 203 mg

Potassium: 143 mg

Phosphorus: 98.2 mg

Ingredients:

Tortillas:
- 8 white corn tortillas
- avocado oil
- sea salt

Beans:
- 2 cups of pinto beans (canned and drained)
- ¼ tsp of chili powder
- ¼ tsp of cumin
- sea salt
- black pepper

Salsa:
- ½ cup of diced tomato
- ¼ cup of diced pineapple
- ¼ cup of cilantro (chopped)
- 3 tbsp of jalapeños (diced) - optional
- 3 tbsp of red onion (diced)
- 1 tbsp of lime juice
- kosher salt
- black pepper

Toppings:
- avocado (sliced)
- lime juice
- cilantro (fresh and chopped)

Directions:

1. Preheat the oven to 425°F and prep two baking sheets with parchment paper.
2. Lightly brush the corn tortillas with oil on both sides and sprinkle with sea salt. Follow this by stacking the baking sheets and lifting one side. Place as many tortillas as you can onto the edge, and lower the top baking sheet. Then, fold the tortillas over the top to form a shell shape with each.
3. Bake the tortillas for 10 to 20 minutes, until they start to turn crisp and light brown, before removing them from a medium heat to cool down.
4. While the tortillas bake, add the pinto beans to a pot and bring to a boil over medium heat, and then lower the heat to simmer the beans until you're ready to add them to the tortilla. Season the beans with cumin, sea salt, and black pepper.
5. Prepare the pineapple salsa by adding all of the remaining ingredients to a small bowl. Toss them to coat, and then taste-test to adjust the flavors as per your preference. Salt can be added for the balance of flavor, lime for acidity, and pineapple for added sweetness.
6. When the tacos are slightly cooked, fill them with pinto beans and the pineapple salsa dressing.

Food-prep tip: Wrap the taco shells in a sheet of parchment paper to seal in freshness for longer. Store them in the refrigerator for up to 3 days.

Moroccan Chicken and Couscous Salad

This chicken and couscous salad is light and quick to make. Containing high-quality protein, this recipe is diabetic-friendly and heart-healthy.

Time: 15 minutes
Serving Size: 6 (2 cups per serving)
Prep Time: 5 minutes
Cook Time: 10 minutes
Nutritional Info:
Calories: 332
Carbs: 51.2 g
Fat: 6.6 g
Protein: 19.6 g
Sodium: 498 mg
Potassium: 322 mg
Phosphorus: 201 mg
Ingredients:
• 2 cups of water + 2 tbsp of water

- 2 cups of chicken (cooked and shredded)
- 1 ½ cups of couscous (uncooked)
- ½ cup of raisins
- ½ cup of orange juice concentrate (undiluted and thawed)
- ⅓ cup of lemon juice
- 2 tbsp of olive oil
- 2 tbsp of cumin
- ½ tbsp of green onions
- ½ tsp of kosher salt
- ¼ tsp of black pepper

Directions:

1. Boil 2 cups of water over medium to high heat in a medium pan. Once boiling, gradually add and stir the couscous and raisins. When it is done cooking, cover it and allow it to stand for 5 minutes, then fluff it with a fork.
2. Combine the orange juice, lemon juice, olive oil, cumin, kosher salt, and black pepper, whisking them together.
3. Combine the couscous mixture with the juice mixture, chicken, and 2 tbsp of water in a bowl. Toss the ingredients to mix, and then garnish them with green onions. Serve hot.

Food-prep tip: Store the chicken and couscous in an airtight container. Keep it in the refrigerator for up to 3 days.

8

Desserts

Frosted Chocolate Cake

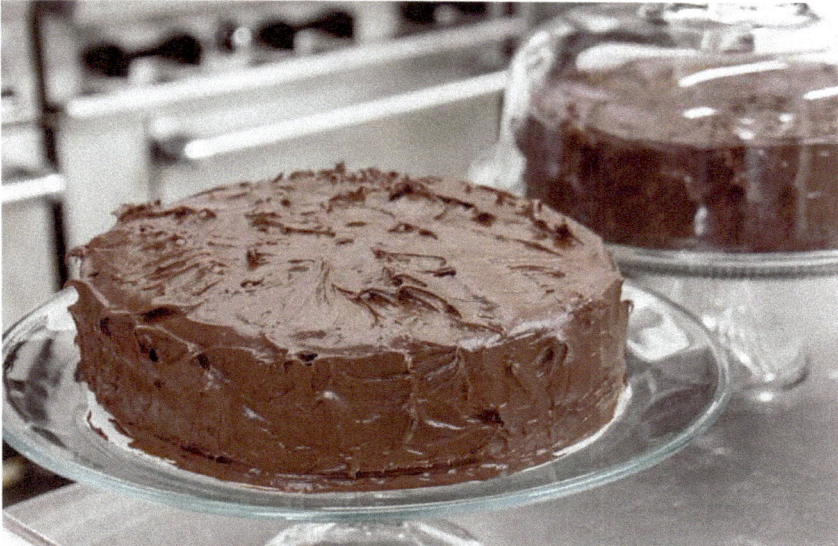

    This cake is decadent and moist without the use of oil. It is also refined-sugar-free, using honey as its only sweetening ingredient. This cake tastes like a cheat meal, but it's low in calories, which means that it's a cleaner and healthier option for dessert.

Time: 1 hour and 32 minutes
Serving Size: 10
Prep Time: 25 minutes
Cook Time: 27 minutes + 40 minutes cooling time
Nutritional Info:
Calories: 292
Carbs: 59 g
Fat: 3 g
Protein: 13 g
Sodium: 305 mg
Potassium: 355 mg
Phosphorus: 215 mg
Ingredients:
Cake:
- 3 eggs
- 2 cups of Greek yogurt
- 2 cups of whole-wheat flour
- 1 cup of maple syrup
- ½ cup of cacao powder
- 1 ½ tsp of baking powder
- 1 tsp of baking soda
- 1 tsp of vanilla extract

Frosting:
- 1 ½ cups of plain Greek yogurt
- ⅓ cup of cacao powder
- ⅓ cup of maple syrup
- ½ tsp of vanilla extract

Directions:

1. For this recipe, you will need 2 cake pans. Place them on 2 large pieces of parchment paper, and circle the pans with a pencil on the outer part of the pans. Use scissors to cut out the shape, place it inside of the cake pan, and spray with cooking spray, including the sides of the pan. Set the cake pans aside for later.
2. Preheat the oven to 350°F.
3. Add the eggs and the cake's maple syrup to a large mixing bowl. Use an electric mixer to beat for 30 seconds. Once done, add in yogurt, baking powder, baking soda, and vanilla. Beat the ingredients with the mixer once more for 30 seconds.
4. Add in the cacao powder, and use a whisk to mix well. Add in the flour, and whisk the mixture once more until you've reached a smooth consistency, but don't overmix it.

5. Divide the batter into two servings for the cake pans, and place them on the bottom rack of the oven for 27 minutes. Once done, test the cakes with a toothpick to see if it is baked through.
6. In the meantime, prepare the frosting by adding the yogurt, cacao powder, maple syrup, and vanilla to a bowl. Whisk the ingredients well and refrigerate the frosting until the cakes are ready to be decorated.
7. Once the cakes are ready, remove them from the oven and allow them to cool first before spreading a ¼ cup of frosting on each.
8. Decorate the cake as you wish and get creative with renal diet-friendly ingredients, such as berries or dark chocolate chips, keeping in mind that any additions will alter the nutritional information. Cut the cake into 10 slices to serve.

Food-prep tip: Store the chocolate cake in the refrigerator in an airtight container for 4 to 5 days. The cake can also be frozen for up to 3 months.

Berry Crumble Squares

These berry squares are inspired by apple crumble, but with berries. It's a low-protein dessert that is also low in calories, and can serve as an ideal treat for someone with a sweet tooth, but who is on a sugar and protein-restricted diet.

Time: 60 minutes
Serving Size: 20
Prep Time: 20 minutes
Cook Time: 40 minutes
Nutritional Info:
Calories: 212
Carbs: 29 g
Fat: 9 g
Protein: 2 g
Sodium: 113 mg
Potassium: 46 mg
Phosphorus: 32 mg
Ingredients:
Crust & topping:
- 1 egg
- zest of 1 small lemon (finely grated)
- 3 cups of flour (all-purpose)
- 1 cup of granulated sugar
- 1 cup of butter (unsalted and cubed)

- 1 tsp of baking powder
- ⅓ tsp of vanilla extract

Berry filling:

- juice of 1 small lemon
- 4 ½ cups fresh berries (chopped)
- ¼ cup of granulated sugar
- 4 tsp of cornstarch

Directions:

1. Using a hand mixer, combine granulated sugar, flour, baking powder, and salt. Add the butter, lemon zest, egg, and vanilla to the mixture. Beat the ingredients at a low speed until the butter is distributed evenly. The mixture should have a crumbly consistency.
2. Add slightly more than half of the mixture to the bottom of the prepped pan, and use the bottom part of a measuring cup to press the dough evenly into the pan.
3. For the filling, gently stir the ingredients until they are well incorporated.
4. Spread the dessert's filling over the crust, and crumble the remaining dough over the berries.
5. Bake the crumble bars for 40 minutes. The top part of the dessert should be light golden brown. Once done, transfer the pan to a rack to cool before cutting it into 20 squares.

Food-prep tip: To store, place the crumble squares in an airtight container in the refrigerator for up to a week.

Banana Peanut Butter Cupcakes

For a low-protein option, these banana peanut butter cupcakes are just the thing to keep you and your family going all week long. Packed with clean ingredients, this dessert is also filled with essential nutrients and offers a nice pick-me-up after a long day at school or work.

Time: 35 minutes
Serving Size: 12
Prep Time: 5 minutes
Cook Time: 30 minutes
Nutritional Info:
Calories: 462.1
Carbs: 43.8 g g
Fat: 29.1 g
Protein: 6.4 g

Sodium: 181.3 mg
Potassium: 248 mg
Phosphorus: 163.3 mg

Ingredients:

Cupcakes:

- 2 bananas (ripe)
- 1 egg
- 1 egg yolk
- 1 ¼ cups of flour (all-purpose)
- ¾ cup of sugar
- ½ cup of butter (unsalted)
- ½ cup of sour cream
- 1 ½ tsp of vanilla extract
- 1 ½ tsp of baking powder
- 1 ½ tsp of vanilla extract
- ½ tsp of baking soda
- ¼ tsp of salt

Frosting:

- 8 oz of cream cheese (packaged)
- 1 ½ cups of powdered sugar
- ½ cup of butter (unsalted)
- ½ cup of peanut butter (smooth)
- ¼ cup of roasted peanuts (chopped and lightly salted)

Directions:

1. Preheat the oven to 350°F and line a standard 12-cup muffin tin with paper liners.
2. Whisk together the flour, baking soda, baking powder, and salt in a medium bowl.
3. Mash the bananas with a fork in a separate medium bowl until they are smooth. Add the cupcake's vanilla extract and sour cream to the bananas.
4. Use the electric mixer to beat the egg, butter and sugar in a large bowl for 3 minutes. The consistency should be light and fluffy. Once done, add the egg yolk and beat until it is well blended. Add the flour mixture, and beat the contents of the once more.
5. Divide the batter evenly among the 12 muffin cups, filling each ¼ full.
6. Bake the cupcakes for 20 minutes. Once done, remove them from the rack and allow them to cool.

7. For the frosting, sift the powdered sugar into a bowl. Then, add in the cream cheese, peanut butter, and butter. Use the electric mixer to beat the mixture until you've reached a smooth consistency.
8. Spread the frosting evenly on top of each of the cupcakes, followed by a handful of chopped peanuts.

Food-prep tip: Store these banana peanut butter muffins in an airtight container in the refrigerator for up to 4 days.

Cream Cheese Pie

This cream cheese pie is just that, creamy! It is low in protein, sodium, potassium, and phosphorus, offering all of the goodness in a dessert minus the guilt.

Time: 40 minutes
Serving Size: 8
Prep Time: 5 minutes
Cook Time: 35 minutes
Nutritional Info:
Calories: 237
Carbs: 35 g
Fat: 9 g
Protein: 4 g
Sodium: 220 mg
Potassium: 162 mg
Phosphorus: 91 mg
Ingredients:
- 8 oz of cream cheese (low-fat)
- 1 9" graham cracker crust (prepped)
- 3 cups of whipped cream (low-sugar, to top)
- 1 ½ cup of raspberries (fresh)
- 1 cup of blueberries (fresh)
- ½ cup of red raspberry preserves (low-sugar)

Directions:

1. For the filling, beat the whipped cream cheese and raspberry preserves with an electric beater on a medium speed, until it reaches a smooth consistency.
2. Fold the whipped cream topping into the cream cheese mixture.
3. Spread the filling layer evenly over the graham cracker crust base, and allow it to chill for 30 minutes in the refrigerator.

4. Before serving the cream pie, arrange the fresh blueberries and raspberries on top.
5. Add a dollop of whipped cream for the topping of the pie.

Food-prep tip: Store the cream pie leftovers in the refrigerator for up to 5 days. Cover it with tin foil or plastic wrap to seal in the pie's freshness.

www.ingramcontent.com/pod-product-compliance
Lightning Source LLC
Chambersburg PA
CBHW060310030426
42336CB00011B/988